CAMBRIDGE CLASSICAL STUDIES

General Editors

D. S. ROBERTSON   F. E. ADCOCK   R. HACKFORTH

W0042127

THE

MEDICAL WRITINGS OF
ANONYMUS LONDINENSIS

THE MEDICAL WRITINGS

OF

ANONYMUS LONDINENSIS

BY

W. H. S. JONES
Litt.D., F.B.A.

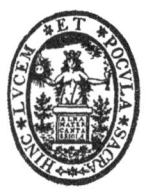

CAMBRIDGE
AT THE UNIVERSITY PRESS

1947

TO THE MEMORY OF

F. M. CORNFORD

CAMBRIDGE UNIVERSITY PRESS
Cambridge, New York, Melbourne, Madrid, Cape Town, Singapore,
São Paulo, Delhi, Dubai, Tokyo, Mexico City

Cambridge University Press
The Edinburgh Building, Cambridge CB2 8RU, UK

Published in the United States of America by Cambridge University Press, New York

www.cambridge.org
Information on this title: www.cambridge.org/9780521170697

© Cambridge University Press 1947

First published 1947
First paperback edition 2010

A catalogue record for this publication is available from the British Library

ISBN 978-0-521-17069-7 Paperback

CONTENTS

PREFACE

When working as Leverhulme Research Fellow on the relations between philosophy and medicine in the ancient world I found it necessary to translate for myself the papyrus known as *Anonymus Londinensis*. On putting my essays together I found that they did not form a homogeneous whole, and it seemed convenient to group most of them round an edition of the Hippocratic *Ancient Medicine*, and to publish separately a translation of *Anonymus* with a few notes and other explanatory matter.

The text of the *editio princeps*, published (with the help of Sir Frederic Kenyon) by Herman Diels in 1893, has been reprinted with only a few changes. The deciphering of such a document is the work of skilled experts, and no scholar without long training in papyrology has any right to emend or criticise the results of those who have devoted a lifetime to this specialised study. The filling in of the gaps in the text and the interpretation of this text are a very different matter, and the mere scholar has a perfect right to form an independent judgment outside the province of the palaeographical experts. Of this right I have availed myself throughout.

The translation is the part of the book to which I have devoted practically my whole attention. The original is full of almost insuperable difficulties, which I have tried to solve by going over it many times, not all at once but after fairly long intervals. Every possible solution has been tried before having recourse to the cheap device of postulating a note-taker's error, although there are many places where such an error seems almost certain, however difficult it may be to put on paper the reasons for this conclusion. Where the text is very mutilated I have usually not ventured either to restore it or to translate the fragments; the few occasions on which I have departed from this rule probably show the wisdom of always faithfully observing it.

A translation of this kind, supplemented by a minimum of comment, may prove useful to students of Greek philosophy who, without a special knowledge of Greek medicine, yet realise its importance for the history of thought. For their sake I have added two supplementary notes, one on the nature of Greek medicine, and one on the peculiar nature of Greek philosophy which led it to introduce its methods into spheres where they were inappropriate. Discussions of many questions raised by *Anonymus* would be endless and for the most part inconclusive. These I have tried to avoid.

I use *"Anonymus"* to denote the text as we now have it, and
"Anonymus" in referring to the person responsible for this text,
whether he was a compiler, a lecturer or a student who took down
lecture notes. There are, I believe, three persons we must try clearly
to distinguish: (1) the scribe, (2) the writer of the text he copied,
and (3) the authority used by this writer. The last may have been an
author in the usual sense, but more probably he was a lecturer. So
when an emendation of the existing text is proposed we must strive
to answer two important questions.

(a)   Was the mistake made by (2), who, misrepresenting (3),
        was faithfully copied by (1)?

(b)   Was the mistake made by (1) who misrepresented (2)?

It is of course not possible always to be sure who made the mistake,
although (2) was probably more often guilty than (1).

In the text I have enclosed between square brackets those parts the
transcription of which is really uncertain, and between daggers those
where the scribe has obviously blundered or repeated himself. Scholars
who wish to know more about the state of the papyrus, the restorations,
contractions, etc. must consult Diels.

While printing Diels' text I have generally translated an emended
text, except in one or two instances where it appeared better to translate
Diels' reading and discuss emendations in a note.

Three debts must be acknowledged. From the edition of Diels
I have taken, with certain modifications, his transcription of the
papyrus, most of his *testimonia* and the *Fragmenta* on (my) pp. 5
and 6. The *Introduction* is indebted to Dr E. T. Withington's article
in *New Chapters in Greek Literature*. But my chief debt is to the late
Professor F. M. Cornford. For three years he guided my work, and
just before his death consented to my dedicating this book to him.
I quote one sentence of the dedication I had prepared: "Alienum
opus tanquam suum curavit."

Even Cornford found some sentences untranslatable, nor could he
offer any solution of the problems presented by the passages so
mutilated that I have been compelled to omit them altogether from
my version.

Professor R. Hackforth has been kind enough to examine a few
places that Cornford left marked with queries.

W. H. S. J.

1946

INTRODUCTION

It was in the *Classical Review* for 1892[1] that Sir Frederic Kenyon announced that in the British Museum was a papyrus of over 1900 lines, a great part of which appeared to be taken from the *Menoneia*, a collection of medical δόξαι mentioned by Galen[2] as attributed by some to Aristotle, but really written by Aristotle's pupil Menon. Kenyon helped the German scholar Hermann Diels to bring out in the following year the *editio princeps*, an invaluable piece of work, which will perhaps never be superseded. The only other work on the *Menoneia* that need be mentioned here is the German translation, with notes, published in 1896 by Heinrich Beckh and Franz Spät. The former was a doctor of philosophy and the latter a doctor of medicine, so that both literary and scientific qualifications were available for the difficult work of producing the *interpretatio princeps*.

The papyrus, according to the experts Kenyon and Diels, is probably of the second century A.D., and it is, according to the same authorities, a copy, made for private use, of an earlier work.

It is about 12 feet long, consisting of 39 columns, each containing 50–60 lines about 3 inches long. In many places it is mutilated or illegible, in many others difficult to decipher; a few lines at the beginning, with the title, are unfortunately lost. The spelling is good, but there are many repetitions and corrections, which suggest that the papyrus is a private copy, not one of an edition. The early date indicated by the character of the papyrus is confirmed by the absence of Galen's name from the authorities mentioned, the latest of whom is Alexander Philalethes, who flourished at the beginning of our era.

Anonymus Londinensis, as the work is now generally called, falls into three distinct, and perhaps unconnected parts:

I–IV, 25	definitions;
IV, 26–XXI, 9	the aetiology of diseases according to various authorities;
XXI, 9–XXXIX, 32	the development of physiology after 300 B.C. from Herophilus to Alexander Philalethes.

---

[1] Pp. 237 foll. "On a Medical Papyrus in the British Museum."
[2] In his commentary on περὶ φύσιος ἀνθρώπου (Kühn, XV. 25). Galen says that another name for the Μενώνεια was Ἰατρικὴ συναγωγή, which is, however, a generic term, "Medical Collection". Galen's words are: πάρεστι σοι τὰς τῆς ἰατρικῆς συναγωγῆς ἀναγνῶναι βίβλους, ἐπιγεγραμμένας μὲν Ἀριστοτέλει, ὁμολογουμένας δὲ ὑπὸ τοῦ Μένωνος, ὃς ἦν μαθητὴς αὐτοῦ, γεγράφθαι, διὸ καὶ Μενώνεια προσαγορεύουσιν ἔνιοι ταυτὶ τὰ βιβλία.

The whole makes a strange mixture, which raises considerable doubt in the reader's mind whether it represents a single work, or two, or possibly even three, separate though slightly connected compilations, perhaps not by the same author.

Chapters I–III with the first nineteen lines of IV contain definitions, often rather confused, of διάθεσις, πάθος, ψυχή, νόσημα, ἀρρώστημα, νόσος and ἀρρωστία. They are of the hair-splitting class, savouring more of the grammarian or logician than of the physician. Little use is made of them in the other sections; in fact the threefold explanation of soul, which is given twice with slight variations, is plainly irrelevant, as the author of the third section declares at the outset that he is not concerned with soul. The author of the first section says that while the first two meanings of soul concern him, the third, which he calls ἐντρέχεια (sic for ἐντελέχεια), does not.

The writer, or lecturer, speaks of certain νεώτεροι, whom he identifies with the Stoics, and also of the τεχνολογία τῶν ἀρχαίων, "whom we also follow". This τεχνολογία too is, in part at least, Stoic, for it refers to the μετριοπάθειαι of the Sage, in the context very like the εὐπάθειαι permitted to the Stoic Wise Man.

The second part, the Menoneia proper, is concerned entirely with the aetiology of diseases. Of the twenty[1] medical authorities quoted, seven[2] were unknown before the discovery of Anonymus. "Aristotle" is quoted as an authority several times, and it is assumed by scholars that he is Menon, whose work, according to Galen, was by general consent written by him although Aristotle was the titular author. Twice[3] Anonymus disagrees with "Aristotle". He is therefore quoting Menon with comments, not merely copying him. It is strange that no reference is made either to Diocles[4] or Praxagoras; stranger still perhaps that the books from which Hippocratic views are extracted are Nature of Man, Diseases I and Breaths, the last of which at any rate no modern scholar would dream of thinking either authentic or genuine. So obviously is Breaths a Sophistic ἐπίδειξις that Wellmann[5] is constrained to believe that "Hippocrates" in Anonymus is not the great physician usually referred to under that name, but his grandson, the son of Thessalus, a possible author of περὶ φυσῶν.

[1] Euryphon, Herodicus, Hippocrates, Alcamenes, Timotheus, Aias (or Abas), Heracleodorus, Herodicus, Minyas, Hippon, Thrasymachus, Dexippus, Phasilas, Aegimius, Plato, Philolaus, Polybus, Menecrates, Petron, Philistion.
[2] These are italicised in the preceding note.
[3] VI. 42–44 and VII. 36.
[4] Unless, as Jäeger thinks, Diocles is post-Aristotelian.
[5] See Hermes, LXI. 333.

The causes of disease are reduced to two classes:

(1) residues (περισσώματα) from food, the cause adopted by the authorities from Euryphon to Aegimius in the above list;

(2) disturbances in the blendings of the elements composing the body, the cause adopted by the others.

Between the two parts, which are of unequal size, comes a long account of Plato's medical views, nearly all of which is taken from *Timaeus*, 69e–86a, though it begins with a discrimination between σύνφθαρσις, μῖξις and διάκρασις, attributed here to Plato, but really Stoic in origin.[1]

The analysis of Plato's medical views which follows is a fairly accurate summary, but in no sort of order, the following being the chief parts of the dialogue treated in turn: 82a, 73a–74a, 69d,e, 80e–81a–c, 74c,d, 74b,c, 74e–75a, 75a–c, 74a,b, 74d, 77c–e, 72c–73a, 45a,b, 69d–70a, 70d–71b, 70c,d, 72c,d, 81e–82e, 84c,d. There is a special difficulty in XVII. 35–43, said to be a quotation (φησίν, l. 36) from Plato, that is, from the *Timaeus*. It is, however, a very free paraphrase of 82d,e. Anonymus, therefore, does not feel bound to quote with verbal accuracy; in some cases at least he (or his teacher) seems to be relying on his memory.

The third section, called by Diels *Eclogae physiologicae* (XXI. 9 to end), is at once the hardest to understand and the most interesting in its subject-matter. It deals with the history of physiology after 300 B.C. from Herophilus to Alexander Philalethes. This department of medical science is called the οἰκονομία of the body, the relation of its receipts to its expenditure. It is a rational and scientific way of regarding the functions of the body, but Anonymus is preoccupied with the assimilation of food and with respiration—two obvious problems which attracted scientific attention earlier than did less obtrusive but equally (or more) essential questions. Beginning with a brief anatomical account of the various parts of the body, the argument goes on to discuss πνεῦμα, nutriment and the various emanations (ἀποφοραί) from the body. Special attention is paid to digestion, to the veins and arteries, and to the invisible "pores". It is not clear, however, what precisely are the theories approved by Anonymus himself.

---

[1] See Stobaeus, *Eclogae*, I. 17, where a similar doctrine is attributed to the Stoics by Arius Didymus. Anonymus appears to be explaining Plato's views by the aid of Stoic τεχνολογία. This passage at least cannot have been derived from the *Menoneia*. The distinction of the words is an interesting but hazy anticipation of the difference between chemical combination and mechanical mixture.

Although the arrangement of the subject-matter improves as the work proceeds—the careless repetitions of the first section are less obvious in the second and third—proof is not required that no section is a redacted work, arranged and prepared for general publication. The scrappiness, slovenly expressions, repetitions and general carelessness speak for themselves, suggesting that the papyrus was intended for the personal use of the writer.

This writer, say the experts, copied some earlier document or documents, which may be called "the original". The nature of this original is a matter of some uncertainty.

(1) If it were a carefully redacted work, one would not expect the copy we possess to contain such glaring and vain repetitions as the accounts of soul in I. 21–27 and II. 7–12.

(2) If it were the work of a professional teacher or similar authority, our copy would probably have been a more finished performance, approximating in literary form to the treatises of Aristotle.

(3) The strange ἐντρέχεια of I. 24 and II. 9 points to an original consisting of lecture-notes taken down by a student in the course of a lecture or lectures.[1] Of course this may be true of the first section without necessarily being true of either the second section or the third. Our copy also appears to have been the work of a young student, as a more advanced scholar would almost certainly have removed most of the existing blemishes.

But a word of caution is necessary. The copy was the work of one scribe, who seems to have produced a paraphrase rather than a copy, but we cannot say that the original also had a single author. Such dissimilar and disconnected parts may have been separate originally, and written out by the copier on one roll for the sake of convenience. So what is probably true of the first section with its tell-tale ἐντρέχεια is not necessarily true of the other two.

Two questions have still to be considered. First, how far does the second part represent Menon, and, secondly, can any plausible guess be made about authorship?

The second part of *Anonymus* (a) is historical, (b) consists of δόξαι and (c) refers, as far as we can see, to no post-Aristotelian authority. All this is consistent with a Menonian origin. On the other hand, the writer must be quoting or paraphrasing, not copying, as he disagrees occasionally with "Aristotle", i.e. Menon, while the δόξαι of Menon

---

[1] Several little touches suggest the lecturer, e.g. the use of the first person and the disrespect shown to thinkers who happen to differ from the speaker (VII. 36: ψεύδεται περὶ τούτων ἀνήρ).

must have had a far wider scope than this second section of *Anonymus*, which is exclusively aetiological. Galen would surely have been less appreciative of Menon's treatise had it been no better than this scrappy fragment, with its disappointing summary of Hippocratic doctrine. We conclude, therefore, that at most the author or lecturer made use of Menon[1] in compiling notes on the causes of disease, and moreover that he did not use him with much care. That such an author should be silent about the views of physicians after 300 B.C. may occasion surprise, but can be reasonably explained in several ways. Perhaps he annotated only the aetiological parts of the *Menoneia*; perhaps a passage may be lost after chapter XX, where, in fact, the papyrus is imperfect.

There are several references to the *Menoneia* in ancient writers, although none of them can be paralleled with anything in *Anonymus*. Galen's remarks are the most informative; the meagreness of the others may be judged from the extracts given below.

ΙΑΤΡΙΚΩΝ ΜΕΝΩΝΕΙΩΝ

FRAGMENTA[2]

I. (Fragm. V. Rose 335 Berlin, 373 Lips.)

Galen (xv. 25 f. K.): καὶ Θεόφραστος δ᾽ ἂν ἐν ταῖς τῶν Φυσικῶν δοξῶν ἐπιτομαῖς τὴν Ξενοφάνους δόξαν, εἴπερ οὕτως εἶχεν, ἐγεγράφει. καί σοι πάρεστιν, εἰ χαίροις τῇ περὶ τούτων ἱστορίᾳ, τὰς τοῦ Θεοφράστου βίβλους ἀναγνῶναι, καθ᾽ ἃς τὴν ἐπιτομὴν ἐποιήσατο τῶν Φυσικῶν δοξῶν, ὥσπερ γε πάλιν εἰ τὰς τῶν παλαιῶν ἰατρῶν δόξας ἐθέλοις ἱστορῆσαι, πάρεστί σοι τὰς τῆς ἰατρικῆς συναγωγῆς ἀναγνῶναι βίβλους, ἐπιγεγραμμένας μὲν Ἀριστοτέλει, ὁμολογουμένας δὲ ὑπὸ τοῦ Μένωνος, ὃς ἦν μαθητὴς αὐτοῦ, γεγράφθαι, διὸ καὶ Μενώνεια προσαγορεύουσιν ἔνιοι ταυτὶ τὰ βιβλία. δῆλον δὲ ὅτι καὶ ὁ Μένων ἐκεῖνος, ἀναζητήσας ἐπιμελῶς τὰ διασῳζόμενα κατ᾽ αὐτὸν ἔτι τῶν παλαιῶν ἰατρῶν βιβλία, τὰς δόξας αὐτῶν ἐκεῖθεν ἀνελέξατο. τῶν δ᾽ ἤδη διεφθαρμένων παντάπασιν, ἢ σῳζομένων μέν, οὐ θεωρηθέντων (?) δ᾽ αὐτῷ, τὰς γνώμας οὐκ ἠδύνατο γράψαι. κατὰ ταῦτ᾽ οὖν τὰ βιβλία χολὴν ξανθὴν ἢ μέλαιναν ἢ φλέγμα στοιχεῖον ἀνθρώπου φύσεως οὐκ ἂν εὕροις οὐδ᾽ ὑφ᾽ ἑνὸς εἰρημένον, αἷμα δὲ καὶ τῶν μεθ᾽ Ἱπποκράτην φαίνονται πολλοὶ μόνον εἶναι νομίζοντες ἐν ἡμῖν, ὥστε καὶ τὴν πρώτην γένεσιν ἡμῶν ἐξ αὐτοῦ γίγνεσθαι, καὶ τὴν μετὰ ταῦτα κατὰ τὴν μήτραν αὔξησιν καὶ ἀποκυηθέντων τελείωσιν.

[1] Or of a doxographer who had made excerpts from his book.
[2] From Diels.

II. (R. 336 B., 374 L.)

Laertius Diogenes, v. 61: γεγόνασι δὲ Στράτωνες ὀκτώ· πρῶτος
Ἰσοκράτους ἀκροατής· δεύτερος αὐτὸς οὗτος· τρίτος ἰατρός, μαθητὴς
Ἐρασιστράτου, ὡς δέ τινες, τρόφιμος,...ἕβδομος ἰατρὸς ἀρχαῖος ὡς
Ἀριστοτέλης φησίν.

III. (R. 337 B., 375 L.)

Plutarch, Quaest. conviv. VIII. 9, 3: καὶ μὴν ἔν γε τοῖς Μενωνείοις
σημεῖον ἡπατικοῦ πάθους ἀναγέγραπται τὸ τοὺς κατοικιδίους μῦς
ἐπιμελῶς παραφυλάττειν καὶ διώκειν.

IV. (R. 339 B., 377 L.)

Caelius Aurelianus, acut. morb. II. 13 (ed. Amman, Amst. 1722, p. 110):
hanc definiens primo De adiutoriis libro Aristoteles sic tradendam credidit.
"pleuritis, inquit, est liquidae materiae coactio sive densatio." nec tamen
disseruit, utrumne totius (quod falsissimum, si quidem phlebotomati aegro-
tantes liquidum sanguinem reddunt), an vero particulae. sed cum hoc
tacuit, necessarium praetermisit.

V. (R. 341 B., 379 L.)

Escolapius, de morbis, p. viii: iracundia irritantur [melancholici] cum
mentis perversitate insaniunt, ut maniaci: in vociferatione solum differunt
Aristotele philosopho testante.

VI. (R. 340 B., 378 L.)

Caelius Aurelianus, chronic. morb. I. 5 (ed. Amman, p. 336): alii frigidis
usi sunt rebus passionis causam ex fervore venire suspicantes, ut Aristoteles
et Diocles.

VII. (R. 338 B., 376 L.)

Pliny, H.N. XXVIII. 74: peculiariter valet potum contra venena quae
data sint e marino lepore, bupresti et aliis, ut Aristoteles tradit, dorycnium;
et contra insaniam quae facta sit hyoscyami potu.

Diels[1] and Ilberg think that the original of Anonymus was a series
of extracts made by a not too cultured student from the Ἀρέσκοντα of
Alexander Philalethes, the latest authority mentioned in the text.

[1] See p. xv: Itaque exarasse haec crediderim adulescentem aliquem medicinae
studiosum, qui in suum sibi usum hanc isagogen describeret. See Hermes, XXVIII.
414.

More interesting is the ingenious theory of Max Wellmann, that the author was Soranus, chief of the eclectic Methodists.[1] The extant works of Soranus show certain similarities of style and language to passages in *Anonymus*, but Wellmann's main argument turns on the quotation from Herophilus at the beginning of the physiological section.[2] It runs thus:

ἁπλᾶ καὶ σύνθετα λαμβάνομεν πρὸς αἴσθησιν καθὼς καὶ Ἡρόφιλος ἐπισημειοῦται, λέγων οὕτως· λεγέσθω δὲ τὰ φαινόμενα πρῶτα, καὶ εἰ μὴ ἔστι πρῶτα.

Now Galen, while criticising the Methodists, makes the following remark:

καί τις ἐπήνεσεν ἐν τούτῳ τὸν Ἡρόφιλον εἰπόντα κατὰ λέξιν οὕτως· λεγέσθω ταῦτ᾽ εἶναι πρῶτα, εἰ καὶ μὴ ἔστι πρῶτα. (*Meth. Med.* 2. 5, Kühn, x. 107.)

Wellmann thinks that the nameless τις must be Soranus, the only Methodist for whom Galen felt any respect, and so refrained from mentioning him by name in a context derogatory to the sect of which he was so distinguished a member. But if τις be Soranus, then he was the author of *Anonymus*, for the sentence beginning with λεγέσθω (XXI. 22) is obviously the one referred to by Galen. The argument is very attractive, although not quite convincing, as the quotation must have been popular with many people of different schools of thought.

If Wellmann's theory be accepted, the third section of *Anonymus* must be a defence of Methodism, which attributed all diseases to constriction and relaxation of invisible πόροι. The Greek text itself, chiefly because of the gaps and imperfections in it, is not quite clear on this point, and the commentator welcomes any possible help in his task of interpretation.

The element of doubt is indeed considerable. Withington[3] points out that Anonymus is critical of all authorities. He spares nobody— Hippocrates, the Empirics, Herophilus, the Erasistrateans, Asclepiades, Alexander, all are attacked. So he must have been, says Withington, either an Eclectic or a Methodist. "It depends on whether he believed in the existence of invisible pores, and attributed disease mainly to their abnormal constriction and relaxation, the doctrine of the Methodic School. He seems at first to take these pores for granted, but we suddenly find him calling an argument of Asclepiades that, because we

[1] See *Hermes*, XL. 580 ff. and LVII. 397 ff. Also, as supplementary to these, LXI. 333.
[2] XXI. 21.   [3] *New Chapters*, pp. 186, 187.

catch a chill after a hot bath, there must be dilated pores which admit the cold air, γελοῖον. It is necessary to prove the existence of pores first. Then follow some mutilated arguments to this effect, and the papyrus concludes φανερὸν τοίγαρτοι ἐκ τούτων καὶ τῶν παραπλησίων, ὡς λόγῳ θεωρητοὶ πόροι εἰσὶν ἐν ἡμῖν καὶ παντὶ ζῴῳ—but it is still not quite certain whether this is some one else's opinion, which he is going to call γελοῖον, or his own, which he is going to make the basis of his pathology on methodic principles."

In short, although invisible pores are constantly discussed, we cannot be sure that the author believed in them. Still less do we know whether, if he believed in pores, he believed that disease is caused by their constriction and relaxation. The only place (XXXVIII. 47) where "open" pores are connected with health—not, by the way, to cause a disease, but only a physical chill—refers to the doctrine of Asclepiades, which is called γελοῖον. Still, in a section dealing with physiology and not with pathology, we might expect a Methodist to be more concerned with the existence of pores and with their normal functions than with their relations to disease. So with some hesitation the Soranus-hypothesis may be accepted as a provisional theory until it can be definitely disproved, or is replaced by one with more extrinsic and intrinsic probability.

The general style of *Anonymus* is similar throughout, except that the worst instances of carelessness occur in the first section. This similarity does not prove that Soranus, even if he be the author of the third section, also composed the other two, for it is a quite possible hypothesis that the copier by paraphrasing gave a similar style to dissimilar originals. Soranus, moreover, may have written the Menon section, but he could scarcely have called himself an adherent of the ἀρχαῖοι, as does the author of the first. The Methodists were a new sect, with radical views about medicine.

The conclusions we may perhaps draw are:

(1) The papyrus is a copy, made by a medical student, of lecture notes also made by a student. (2) It may represent several lectures, the lecturer using the συναγωγή of Menon for one of them. (3) The lecturer corresponding to the third section was probably Soranus, who possibly was responsible for the second also but not for the first. (4) Another source used by the lecturer (or lecturers) may have been the Ἀρέσκοντα of Alexander Philalethes.

ADDITIONAL NOTES

(A) Δύναμις in scientific writings

The meaning of δύναμις in Greek science is very different from the Aristotelian "potentiality". Cornford[1] calls δυνάμεις the properties of bodies considered as having the power to act and be acted upon, e.g. hotness is the property of fire that is manifest when fire makes something hot or causes in sentient things a sensation of heat. "Property", "quality" or "characteristic" are possible but partial equivalents in many cases; what is lacking in these renderings is that a δύναμις always belongs to a thing's real nature. It is, in fact, the active side of a φύσις. "Essence" or "essential characteristic" are thus also possible equivalents, but even these fail to suggest the idea of force or action associated with the word. In *Nature of Man*, v, occur the phrases τὴν ἰδέην τε καὶ τὴν δύναμιν and ἔχει δύναμίν τε καὶ φύσιν τὴν ἑωυτοῦ, showing the close relationship of δύναμις to the scientific terms denoting reality. But it is in *Regimen* I. iii that the most instructive example is given: "Now all living creatures, including man, are composed of two things, differing in power, but complementary in their use, namely fire and water....Now the power (δύναμιν) that each possesses is that fire can (δύναται) move all things always, while water can nourish all things always." In other words, according to this writer, the δυνάμεις of fire and water are force and nutritiveness. *Ancient Medicine* recognises a number of δυνάμεις, that of fire being heat. This, and the traditional opposites, the writer considers of little importance to human health;[2] far more important are a number (how many is not specified) of other δυνάμεις, the sweet, the bitter, the astringent and so on, which, if strong (ἰσχυρά) and unblended (ἄκρητα), cause disease, while a κρᾶσις of them results in health. He reduces the whole art of medicine to the maintenance of such a κρᾶσις by strict attention to regimen. *Regimen* I[3] speaks of "powers" of sea, moon and stars, meaning their essential functions, while *Ancient Medicine* mentions τὴν τοῦ ἀνθρώπου φύσιν τε καὶ δύναμιν.[4]

[1] *The Cosmology of Plato*, p. 53.
[2] Ch. xvi. See also xiv and xv. Particularly instructive are xv (end) and xix: τἆλλα ὅσα κακοπαθεῖ ὁ ἄνθρωπος πάντα ἀπὸ δυναμίων γίνεται.
[3] Ch. x.
[4] Ch. iii. The δύναμις ἀνθρώπου would be human nature in its widest sense, not as a mere passive reality, but as affecting its environment in certain ways. Certain effects in us, the result of our reactions to contact with a human being, correspond to that human being's δύναμις.

Although the argument of *Ancient Medicine* is clearly and fully set forth—δύναμις, ἰσχυρός, ἰσχυρῶς are repeatedly explained throughout the discussion—yet a modern reader experiences a difficulty in completely understanding it because in the *Corpus Hippocraticum* "the hot", "the cold" and many other powers, while no longer regarded as bodies, were not yet merely qualities. Even in the post-Aristotelian *Anonymus* some confusion of thought may be felt. Perhaps the clearest exposition is that found in Plato's *Phaedrus*, 270 c, d, where Hippocrates is cited with approval as holding the view that to discover the φύσις of a thing its δύναμις (or δυνάμεις if it be complex), that is its power of ποιεῖν or παθεῖν, must be examined to find its relation to other things. In other words, realities can manifest themselves to our senses in certain ways which represent their "powers". Possibly the best and most informative English equivalent for δύναμις is "property". Of course, even in a scientific work, the word may have its ordinary meaning, "power" or "force". See J. Souilhé, *Étude sur le terme* δύναμις, pp. 31–57 and A. Keus, *Ueber philosophische Begriffe und Theorien in den Hippokrateischen Schriften*, pp. 46–58.

(B)   Πνεῦμα

There are few words used by Greek thinkers more interesting than those roughly equivalent to "air", especially πνεῦμα. They are three in number (ἀήρ, φῦσα, πνεῦμα). The first of these was perhaps the most general in meaning, although in Ionic, and therefore in most scientific writings, it meant "mist", or at least the lower atmosphere. The second (φῦσα) is limited by the author of περὶ φυσῶν to air in the body (that we should perhaps call "gas"), πνεῦμα to air outside the body, but there cannot have been a strict consistency in the use of such words, the Hippocratic writer himself using indifferently, for air outside the body, πνεῦμα and ἀήρ. In the pre-scientific stage of chemistry all "gases" were looked upon as "air" with specific qualities to give them individuality. In the same way, subconsciously at least, all liquids were regarded as different kinds of "water". But φῦσα, and to a much greater degree πνεῦμα, implied motion; πνέω was used of wind, εἰσπνέω and ἐκπνέω of breathing.

The obvious connection between air and life could not escape the notice of the Greeks, for without air animals cannot live. Nay, the author of περὶ φυσῶν (ch. III) notices that even fish must breathe, and assures us that wind is food for fire, and without air fire cannot live.

So πνεῦμα was associated with ideas of vitality and motion, as much as was fire, if not more so. In fact the two were often combined, special virtues being assigned to warm or even fiery breath. The πνεῦμα of Erasistratus discussed in the physiological section of *Anonymus* was a life-giving gas circulating in the arteries, as opposed to the doctrine of those who looked upon πνεῦμα as the cooler of ἔμφυτον θερμόν.[1] The confusing theories of the Pneumatists agreed in this, that πνεῦμα was essential, owing to some special quality in it, to true vitality. Hence arose what Clifford Allbutt calls the "pathetic quest" for this vital element, which resulted finally, on the physical side, in the discovery of oxygen. On the spiritual side we have the λόγος doctrine of the Stoics and the ἅγιον πνεῦμα of St John.

It is, of course, impossible for the translator to be quite consistent. He has to choose the English equivalent which suits best each separate context.

(C) Περίσσωμα and σύντηξις

The modern physiologist is often at a loss if asked to find equivalents for old physiological terms. For the whole group of ideas, with the help of which a present-day professor explains the bodily functions, is very different from that which directed the mind of Hippocrates or of Galen. Not only was physiology imperfectly understood, but also many things now known to be abstract qualities were then regarded as corporeal substances.

Περίσσωμα is a case in point. Defined by Aristotle as τὸ τῆς τροφῆς ὑπόλειμμα,[2] it has by many been translated "superfluity". Perhaps "residue" would be a better word, as "superfluity" suggests excess, but περίσσωμα a useless remainder. A ton of apples would be a superfluity of digestible material for a man; from even one apple there would be an indigestible περίσσωμα.

Aegimius of Elis[3] held that such a περίσσωμα underwent σύντηξις (colliquescence). Then it was either excreted by the normal channels or secreted in the form of juices circulating in the body. Apparently deficient σύντηξις would result in πλῆθος τῶν περισσωμάτων, thus being a cause of disease.

But a word of caution is necessary. Aristotle uses both these terms, but with refinements and much elaboration. He recognises e.g. "useful" as well as "useless" περισσώματα, whereas in *Anonymus*

---

[1] There seems, however, to be some doubt how Erasistratus regarded the function of respiration. See Clifford Allbutt, *Greek Medicine at Rome, s.v.* in the index. Especially important are pp. 150 and 258.

[2] *Gen. Anim.* 724b 26.　　　　　[3] *Anonymus*, XIII. 26 ff.

the term means little more than the unabsorbed parts of food, being roughly divided into (*a*) *excreta* and (*b*) certain fluids circulating in the body.

The probable explanation of these differences is that Aristotle took the material collected by his pupil Menon, and elaborated those parts which best suited his own views and objects.

(D)   κενὸς ἀθροῦς τόπος.

In several places (XXVI. 48 c; XXVII. 6, 7, 29, 38) occurs the phrase κενὸς ἀθροῦς τόπος, or ὁ κενὸς ἀθροῦς. The phrase, apparently first used by Erasistratus, is connected with the view, which seems to have originated with Straton, that Nature abhors a vacuum (*horror vacui*). The Atomists postulated void, τὸ κενόν, in order to explain motion. The idea of empty space without any atoms disseminated in it does not seem to have troubled early thinkers. But with the notion that a vacuum tends to fill itself from neighbouring matter came the need to distinguish void filled with disseminated atoms from void not so filled, and the adjective ἀθροῦς was used for that purpose. Perhaps τὸ κενόν = "void" and ἀθροῦς κενὸς τόπος = "a vacuum" or "empty space". Diels (pp. 1 and 81) refers to his article "Über das physikalische System des Straton" in *Sitzungsberichte der Berl. Akad.* 1893, pp. 101–27.

(E)   Analysis of I 1–IV. 17

Preliminary Classification of Affections (πάθη).

I. 1–14. The definition of πάθος includes the term διάθεσις, in this context that of a δύναμις, either ζωτική, σωματική or ψυχική.

[The first we should now call "life", the subject of physiology and bio-chemistry; the second is the subject of anatomy, and the third, almost "consciousness", is the subject of psychology.] These διαθέσεις may be: (*a*) πάθη κατὰ κίνησιν, all κινήματα being such; (*b*) πάθη κατὰ σχέσιν, e.g. paralysis, etc.

15–27. Some πάθη are ψυχικά, others σωματικά; under the term "bodily" we may comprise all σωματικαὶ δυνάμεις and ἡ ζωτικὴ δύναμις, in contrast to ψυχή, thus getting:

(*a*) σωματικὰ πάθη, i.e. abnormal conditions, physical or physiological;

(*b*) ψυχικὰ πάθη, i.e. abnormal conditions of the soul, which is used in three senses: ἡ τῷ ὅλῳ σώματι παρεσπαρμένη [the psychical aspect of ἡ ζωτικὴ δύναμις]; (2) τὸ λογιστικὸν μόριον [the mind]; (3) ἡ ἐντρέχεια [a metaphysical concept that does not concern physicians].

26–40. With the other kinds of soul, especially with τὸ λογιστικόν, physicians are concerned, for it is in this in particular that arise ψυχικὰ πάθη, whether antecedent (προηγούμενα) or consequential (τὰ κατ' ἐπακολούθημα).

Examples of ψυχικὰ πάθη that are προηγούμενα κατὰ κίνησιν: δεισιδαιμονία, λύπη, φόβος, φιλαργυρία; of προηγούμενα ἐν σχέσει examples are κάρος and λήθαργος.

Of σωματικὰ πάθη an example is πυρετός, an antecedent affection of the body producing in the soul the consequential affection of delirium, a πάθος ἐν κινήσει. Of affections ἐν σχέσει examples are παράλυσις, κάρος, etc.

A paragraph repeating some of the above.

I. 40–II. 4. Some πάθη are σωματικά, others ψυχικά. (a) σωματικά are always προηγούμενα and closely bound up with the power of life; ψυχικά are bound up with the "soul that is in the body". So these, "life" and "soul in the body", are powers in a special sense. [Though carefully to be distinguished from each other (I. 19–21), both are links between body and soul. E.g. fever, a σωματικὸν πάθος, starts in the body, but has a consequential effect upon τὸ λογιστικόν, which it reaches through the agency of ἡ ζωτική; while φόβος, a προηγούμενον πάθος κατὰ κίνησιν of τὸ λογιστικόν (I. 29–31), affects the body through the "soul that is in the body", but does not produce a consequential σωματικὸν πάθος.]

II. 4–III. 7. Revision with elaboration of ψυχικὸν πάθος.

II. 4–12. A ψυχικὸν πάθος is a διάθεσις ψυχῆς κατὰ κίνησιν ἢ σχέσιν—for ψυχή too is a δύναμις. There are three meanings of ψυχή: ἡ ὅλη ψυχή, τὸ μέρος τὸ λογιστικόν, αὐτὴ ἡ ἐντρέχεια. When we speak of "psychic affections" the first two are involved.

12–22. Psychic affections are either κατὰ φύσιν or παρὰ φύσιν. So the full description of a psychic affection is διαθετικὸν ψυχῆς κατὰ κίνησιν ἢ κατὰ σχέσιν, κατὰ φύσιν ἢ παρὰ φύσιν. This is the terminology of our own sect, οἱ ἀρχαῖοι, who permit the Sage to feel μετριοπάθειαι.

22–30. The Stoics, οἱ νεώτεροι, hold that no ψυχικὸν πάθος is κατὰ φύσιν.

II. 31–III. 7. But we hold that, e.g. μνήμη and διαλογισμός are psychic affections κατὰ φύσιν, while ἀμνημοσύνη and ἀλογία are παρὰ φύσιν. The most generic of these according to "the ancients" are ἡδονή and ὄχλησις; according to the Stoics ἡδονή, ἐπιθυμία, φόβος and λύπη. III. 7–IV. 17. A discussion of σωματικὰ πάθη with elaborate classification of the various species.

(F) Physicians and Philosophers referred to in *Anonymus*

Names in italics are otherwise unknown

Abas or *Aias*

Aegimius of Elis

A contemporary, perhaps a younger contemporary, of Hippocrates, who wrote περὶ παλμῶν. See Galen, VIII. 498, 752.

Alcamenes of Abydos

Alexander Philalethes

A pupil of Asclepiades, who flourished at the beginning of our era and wrote Ἀρέσκοντα, which some think a source used by Anonymus. Diels in *Hermes*, XXVIII. 414.

"Aristotle"

The name used by Anonymus when he is referring to Menon's work.

Asclepiades

A fashionable physician who went to Rome in 91 B.C. He introduced a new theory of disease based on atomism. The body was thought to be composed of atoms, with pores between them, diseases being ascribed to changes in the relations of atoms and pores, especially to the blocking up of pores. Asclepiades was nicknamed "Wine-giver" (οἰνοδότης).

Dexippus of Cos

A pupil of Hippocrates who flourished in the earlier part of the fourth century B.C. His doctrines as given in XII. 9 ff. have some interesting parallels in the Hippocratic *Corpus*. See p. 18. See also *Suidas*, s. v., and Galen, I. 144, XV. 478, 703, 744 and XI. 182.

Erasistratus

A slightly younger contemporary of Herophilus, who came to Alexandria in the first part of the third century B.C. A physiologist who rejected the humoral pathology, he substituted a doctrine of πνεῦμα, the action of which he regarded as purely mechanical. He reverted to the Hippocratic view that medicine is but a branch of dietetics, and thus rejected bleeding and all but the mildest drugs. See J. F. Dobson in *Proc.* of Roy. Soc. of Med. 1927.

Euryphon

The reputed author of *Cnidian Sentences* (Galen, XVII. A 886) and of περὶ διαίτης ὑγιεινῆς (XV. 455). Some have felt inclined to attribute to him περὶ διαίτης (Galen, VI. 473), and also περὶ νούσων II (Galen, XVII. A 888, Littré, I. 47, 363). According to Caelius Aurelianus (*De morbis chronicis*, II. 10, p. 390) he was aware of the difference between arteries and veins, knowing that the former too contain blood. He founded the Cnidian School.

Heracleodorus
Herodicus (of Cnidos)

Little is known of this physician. Besides *Anonymus*, IV. 41 ff., see Galen, XVII. B 99 and Plato, *Gorgias*, 448 b.

Herodicus (of Selymbria)

Famous for his over-exercising his patients. He is mentioned by Plato, who seems to have felt some dislike of the man and of his methods. See the *Testimonia* to IX. 20. A fifth-century παιδοτρίβης who applied himself to medicine. Probably not the Herodicus mentioned among the teachers of Hippocrates.

Herophilus

A skilled anatomist of the fourth and third centuries B.C. He worked in the medical school at Alexandria, paid attention to pulses and studied carefully the brain. He is said to have conducted *post-mortem* examinations. See J. F. Dobson, *Proc.* of Roy. Soc. of Med. 1925.

Hippon of Croton

A belated follower of Thales who flourished in the time of Pericles. See *Hermes*, XXVIII. 420 and Zeller, *Pre-Socratic Philosophy*, I. 281–283 (Eng. tr.).

"Hippocrates"

Anonymus assigns to "Hippocrates" such un-Hippocratic works that some scholars doubt whether he refers to the "great" Hippocrates. See p. 2 and note H.

Menecrates

A Syracusan who spent some time at the court of King Philip. See Suidas *s.v.*, Aelian, *V.H.* XII. 51; *Hermes*, XXVIII. 416 ff. Beckh and Spät, pp. 95–98 and O. Weinreich, *Menekrates Zeus und Salmoneus*.

Ninyas the Egyptian

Petron of Aegina

Perhaps the Petronas of Galen (I. 144, XV. 436). He flourished after Hippocrates but before Herophilus. Mentioned by Celsus (III. 9). See Beckh and Spät, p. 98.

Phaselas of Tenedos

Philistion

A famous physician who seems to have had much influence on Plato. Born in Sicily or S. Italy, he became tutor to Chrysippus of Cnidos and therefore belongs to the fourth century. Thought by some to have written περὶ διαίτης ὑγιεινῆς (Galen, XV. 455). See M. Wellmann, *Die Fragmente der Sikelischen Ärŧte*, pp. 109–116.

Philolaus of Croton

The teacher of Simmias and Cebes, young friends of Socrates. He was known as a Pythagorean philosopher rather than as a physician. His view that our bodies are composed of τὸ θερμόν can be paralleled in περὶ σαρκῶν (ch. 11), while in his aetiology of disease he reverted to the humoral pathology (*Anonymus*, XVIII. 30). See *Hermes*, XXVIII. 417.

Plato

Nearly all the theories attributed by Anonymus to Plato come from the later sections of the *Timaeus*.

Polybus

The pupil and son-in-law of Hippocrates, and one of the founders of Dogmatism. Anonymus (XIX. 9) attributes the doctrine of περὶ φύσιος ἀνθρώπου IV to Polybus, but (VII. 15) that of ch. IX to "Hippocrates". Galen (XV. 11 and 175, XVI. 3) gives some information about him, being inclined to attribute to him both περὶ φύσιος ἀνθρώπου and περὶ διαίτης ὑγιεινῆς.

Thrasymachus of Sardis

Timotheus of Metapontum

(G) Passages from the *Corpus Hippocraticum* illustrating
Anonymus XIV–XX

(1) "Both men and women have in their bodies four forms (ἰδέας)
of the moist, from which diseases arise, except such cases as are the
result of violence. These forms are phlegm, blood, bile and watery
humour (ὕδρωψ)." [*Diseases* IV, 32 (Littré VII. 542).]
ὕδρωψ. Littré translates "l'eau", and in chapter 33 both ὕδρωψ and
ὕδωρ occur with apparently the same meaning, and a like interchange
occurs in chapter 37. Perhaps the writer wished to choose a term
which did not exclude watery fluids such as spittle, mucus and serum.
The question whether ὕδρωψ has any particular meaning different from
ὕδωρ becomes more doubtful when we take account of *Generation* 3,
a passage which, whatever its origin, is closely connected with chapter 32
of *Diseases* IV. It runs:

(2) "There are four forms of the moist—blood, bile, water (ὕδωρ)
and phlegm. For this is the number of forms that man has innate in
himself, and from them diseases arise. I have discussed these already,
and shown why diseases and their crises (διακρίσιες) originate from
them." [Littré, VII. 474.]

Unless this chapter be an insertion, it is plain that *Generation* was
written after *Diseases* IV. The latter also seems to imply that the four
ἰδέαι of moisture exhaust the constituents of the body; the former says
that the seed comes "from all the body, the hard parts, the soft parts
and from all the moisture in the body".

(3) Two works in the *Corpus* reduce the causes of disease, though
not necessarily the constituents of the body, to bile and phlegm.

(a) *Diseases* I, a separate work unconnected with the other books
II, III and IV, has the following passage:

"All diseases arise from the internal causes of bile and phlegm, and
from the external causes of fatigue, wounds, excessive heat, cold, dryness or moisture. Bile and phlegm are congenital, and are always
present in the body to a greater or less amount. They cause diseases,
the secondary causes being food, drink, excessive heat or excessive
cold." [Chapter 2 (Littré, VI. 142).]

(b) *Affections* is a description of common diseases written, as the
first chapter says, to give the layman such information as will enable
him and the practitioner to understand each other. After the opening
sentences the author goes on thus:

"All diseases arise in men through bile and phlegm. Bile and phlegm cause diseases when in the body they are affected by excess of dryness, moisture, heat or cold. Phlegm and bile are so affected as the result, not only of heat and cold, but also of food and drink, of fatigue and wounds, of smell, hearing, sight or venery. The occasion of their being affected is when any of the aforesaid influences act upon the body unseasonably, or contrary to habit, or in excess and with violence, or deficiently and weakly. All the diseases of men come from these causes. About these matters the layman ought to know all that it is reasonable to expect a layman to learn. As to the knowledge, prescriptions and operations of the practitioner, the layman ought to be able to co-operate by a kind of appreciation both of what is said and of what is being done." [Chapter I (Littré, vi. 208).]

The second passage is an enlargement and refinement of the first, and the doctrine it contains seems to have been not uncommon among doctors of the late fifth and early fourth centuries B.C. The mutilated beginning, for instance, of the seventh column of *Anonymus Londinensis* mentions the view that diseases arise from bile and phlegm when acted upon by heat and cold,[1] the next sentence suggesting that the writer attributed such a doctrine to "Hippocrates". Later, in XII, speaking of Dexippus of Cos, a pupil of Hippocrates, the writer says that diseases are caused "from the powers of bile and phlegm arising in a part of the body or the whole, these being stirred up, not of themselves, but through many unseasonable partakings of nutriment. These things cause disease, he says, by reason of their quantity, their position and their form, and he considers that change takes place also through excess of anything—of heat, of cold, or of similar things."

The same writer in XI attributes to the otherwise unknown Thrasymachus of Sardis the theory that the cause of disease is the changing of blood under the action of cold or heat into phlegm, bile or pus ($\sigma\epsilon\sigma\eta\pi\acute{o}s$). Philolaus (XVIII) made bile, blood and phlegm the causes of disease, but considered heat the stuff from which our bodies are made. Again, in XIX Menecrates surnamed Zeus is said to have analysed the human body into four elements, two (blood and bile) hot, and two (breath and phlegm) cold. When these are in harmony ($\epsilon\mathring{v}\kappa\rho\acute{o}\tau\omega s$ $\delta\iota\alpha\kappa\epsilon\iota\mu\acute{e}\nu\omega\nu$) the result is health; when they are not in harmony, the result is disease.

---

[1] Petron of Aegina (*Anon.* XX) is said to have made these opposites elemental, and to have held that abnormalities in their blending are one cause of diseases.

The last doctrine approaches very near to the traditional view of the four humours, blood, phlegm, yellow bile and black bile, as set forth in the famous *Nature of Man*:

"The body of man has in itself blood, phlegm, yellow bile and black bile; these make up the stuff (φύσις) of his body, and through these he feels pain or enjoys health. Now he enjoys the most perfect health when these constituents are duly proportioned to one another in respect of compounding, power and bulk, that is, when the mixture is perfect." [Chapter IV.]

Philistion held a similar view, except that he took the traditional elements to be the components of the body.

These theories may be divided into two classes:

(1) those that make the "humours" elemental;
(2) those that do not do so, or leave the question open.

The former include *Diseases* IV and *Generation*, where the four humours concerned are called "really existent forms" (ἰδέαι) of the moist, Thrasymachus, who held blood to be elemental but not the others, Menecrates, who calls blood, bile, πνεῦμα and phlegm στοιχεῖα, and *Nature of Man*. To these must possibly be added Dexippus. Of the others, Philolaus and Petron certainly, *Diseases* I, *Affections* and *Anonymus* VII (*initium*) probably, looked upon humours as not elemental. Philistion appears to have abandoned the humoral pathology altogether.

To regard the humours as elemental was not a popular view with philosophers after Anaxagoras. It seems to have been confined to the physicians, being especially attractive to the Coan school. Philolaus, Philistion and Plato would have none of it.

(H) Menon on Hippocrates

For many years after the discovery of *Anonymus* historians of medicine were very disappointed with the account of Hippocrates as given in V. 35–VII. 40.[1] It appears to be a not very accurate summary of the Sophistic dissertation *Breaths*, taken chiefly from the seventh chapter, and followed by a grumble of the lecturer (compiler), who says that "Aristotle" (that is, Menon) gives one account of Hippocrates, but Hippocrates himself says something different (VI. 42–45 and VII. 37–40). There is given in Chapter VII what is said to be the

[1] A probable, but unprovable, hypothesis, which would remove many difficulties from the Menonian section, is that Anonymus used, not Menon's work, but an imperfect *précis* of it.

real Hippocratic doctrine, taken chiefly from *Diseases*, I, ii, and *Nature of Man*, iv and ix.[1]

During the past ten years the opinion has been gaining ground that *Anonymus* V. 35–VI. 42, together with Plato *Phaedrus*, 270 c, d, are the only reliable testimony for the doctrine of the historical Hippocrates, not one of the works in the *Corpus Hippocraticum* being supported by really reliable evidence.[2] It is argued that Hippocrates won a great name for himself by his practical skill, and perhaps by writings which have since perished. Then, in the Alexandrine age, when great libraries were being formed, anonymous works collected from various sources were ascribed to the most famous of all physicians, or to his school, in order to enhance their value.

The books in the *Corpus* are all anonymous. Many of them are demonstrably not from the hand of Hippocrates nor inspired by Coan teaching; the commentators, from Bacchius to Galen, have rejected many, and marked many others as doubtful.

When the region of uncertainty is so great, the sceptic who rejects all post-Aristotelian testimony has little difficulty in making out a plausible, if not a probable case. But if this view be correct, we know little about Hippocrates. Plato tells us something about Hippocrates' method of studying the φύσις of man, though the passage in the *Phaedrus* is short, and not free from ambiguities. Menon says that Hippocrates supposed the origin of diseases to be φῦσαι arising from περισσώματα of food. All this is interesting, and of some importance; but it is scarcely enough to account for the title of "the Great", which Hippocrates had won by the time of Aristotle (*Politics* 1326a).

The question of authorship is not likely ever to be finally settled. On the other hand, we do possess the *Corpus*, of which several books are in a true sense great achievements, with consistent doctrines inspired by all that is best in the scientific spirit. The Hippocratic problem, like the Homeric problem, cannot take from us our heritage.

For a fuller discussion of the question see *Hippocrates and the Corpus Hippocraticum* by W. H. S. Jones in the *Proceedings* of the British Academy for 1945.

---

[1] Yet in XIX chapters III and IV are ascribed to Polybus, to whom Aristotle himself (*Historia animalium* III 3) ascribes the chapter (XI) on the veins.

[2] The chief exponent is L. Edelstein. See his *Nachträge* (Hippokrates) to Paulys *Realencyclopädie, Problemata* IV, περὶ ἀέρων etc., *The Genuine Works of Hippocrates* (*Bulletin of the History of Medicine*, 1939) and a review of M. Pohlenz. *Hippokrates und die Begründung der wissenschaftlichen Medizin*, in *American Journal of Philology*, April 1940.

BIBLIOGRAPHY

F. G. Kenyon in *Classical Review*, 1892, pp. 237 ff.

Hermes, XXVIII. 406–434 (H. Diels).

Hermes, XL. 580 ff. (Max Wellmann).

Hermes, LVII. 397 ff. (Max Wellmann).

Hermes, LXI. 333 (Max Wellmann).

H. Diels. *Anonymi Londinensis ex Aristotelis Iatricis Menoniis et aliis Medicis Eclogae*, Berlin 1893.

F. v. Oefele. *All. med. Centralzeitung* (Nr 11), 1895, *Aerztlich. Rundschau* (Nr 17), 1895.

H. Beckh and F. Spät in *Janus* for 1896.

H. Beckh und F. Spät. *Anonymus Londinensis.* German translation, Berlin 1897.

E. T. Withington in *New Chapters in the History of Greek Literature*, second series, edited by J. U. Powell and E. A. Barber, Oxford 1929.

L. Edelstein (1) περὶ ἀέρων *und die Sammlung der Hippokratischen Schriften*, Berlin 1931.

    (2) Paulys *Realencyclopädie*, Nachträge (Hippokrates) pp. 1290–1343, Stuttgart n.d.

    (3) *The Genuine Works of Hippocrates*, in *Bulletin of the History of Medicine*, Vol. VII, No. 2, 1939.

ABBREVIATIONS

D. = H. Diels in his *editio princeps*.

K. = Sir Frederic Kenyon, as referred to by Diels.

L. = Littré's edition of Hippocrates.

P. = the text of the papyrus.

B. and S. = the German translation by Beckh and Spät.

The text is a reprint of that of Diels. A few obvious slips and dittographies, often corrected by the copyist himself, have also been omitted, while a few printer's errors etc. have been corrected. Square brackets [ ] mean that the text is very uncertain, while daggers †† mark the scribe's errors, repetitions, etc. The columns of the papyrus are given in Roman numerals in the margin of both text and translation, and the chapters of B. and S. are given in Arabic numerals in the margin of the translation only. The stars (text and translation) mean space for a letter or letters.

ANONYMI LONDINENSIS IATRICA

I ......νοντας ἐν τῶι τοῦ π.........
...... ν πρὸς τῶν ἀρχαίων κ.....με-
......σιν καὶ ἐπίτασιν καὶ ἄνεσιν ἀνα
......ένην. μάλιστα γὰρ συμφερόμε-
5 θα καὶ αὐτοὶ τοῖς ἀρχαίοις. καὶ τί μέν ἐστιν διάθεσις καὶ ποίαν κομίζομεν ἐν τῶι ὅρωι,
ἀπεδείξαμεν· διάθεσις δυνάμεως ἡσδήπο-
τε, εἴτε τῆς ζωτικῆς εἴτε τῆς σωμα-
τικῆς εἴτε τῆς ἐν τοῖς σώμασι
10 ἐνούσης ψυχικῆς, κατὰ κείνησιν
ἢ σχέσιν, κατὰ κείνησιν μὲν πάντα τὰ
ἐν ἡμῖν κεινήματα πάθη κατὰ
κείνησίν ἐστιν, κατὰ σχέσιν δὲ παράλυσις, λήθαργος, κάρος, τὰ τούτοις ἐγγύς.
15 τούτων δὲ κειμένων δεῖ γινώσκειν ὡς τῶν παθῶν τὰ
μέν φασιν εἶναι ψυχικά, τὰ δὲ σωματικά, σωματικὰ λαμβάνοντες τὰ περὶ τὴν
ζωτικὴν δύναμιν λαμβανόμενα,
[τάς τε ἄ]λλας δυνάμεις ἀντιδιαστέλ-
20 [λοντες κ]αὶ τὴν ζωτικὴν δύναμιν
τῆι ψυχῆι. ψυχὴ δὲ λέγεται τριχῶς·
ἥ τε τῶι ὅλωι σώματι παρεσπαρμένη καὶ τὸ μόριον τὸ λογιστικὸν
καὶ ἔτι ἡ ἐντρέχεια. * καὶ τῆς μὲν ἐντρε-
25 χείας ἐπὶ τοῦ παρόντος οὐ χρῄζομεν,
τῶν δὲ ἄλλων δύο σημαινομένων,

Testimonia.

7. Galen (x. 51 K.): πάντες γοῦν σχεδὸν οἱ ἀπὸ τῆς ἀμεθόδου τε καὶ
μανιώδους ταύτης αἱρέσεως τὴν μὲν ὑγείαν εὐστάθειαν τῶν κατὰ φύσιν
ἐνεργειῶν εἶναί φασι καὶ ἰσχύν, τὴν δὲ νόσον οὐκέτι βλάβην ἐνεργείας καὶ
ἀσθένειαν, ἀλλ' οἱ μὲν διάθεσίν τινα σώματος, οἱ δὲ σῶμά πως διακείμενον
(cf. x. 54).

---

1. According to D. the general sense was: περιλαμβάνοντες ἐν τῷ
τοῦ πάθους ὅρῳ καὶ τὴν πρὸς τῶν ἀρχαίων κομιζομένην κρᾶσιν, καὶ
ἐπίτασιν καὶ ἄνεσιν ἀνὰ λόγον δεχομένην.
19, 20. The additions are very uncertain.

MEDICAL WRITINGS OF
ANONYMUS LONDINENSIS

INTRODUCTORY DEFINITIONS

I ...comprising in the definition of "affection" the term "blending" also, in the sense given to it by the ancients, that allows a component to be strong proportionally to the weakness of another. For we too are in full agreement with the ancients. What a condition is, and what kind of condition we mean in the definition, we have explained. It is a condition of a power of whatever kind it may be, either the power of life or of the body or of the soul that is in the body, being either kinetic or static; (a) kinetic: all movements in us are kinetic affections; (b) static are paralysis, coma, torpor and similar affections.

This having been established, we must learn that of affections some are said to be psychological, others bodily, including as bodily all those included under the power of life, and distinguishing the powers, especially the power of life, from the soul. The word "soul" is used in three senses: (1) the soul that pervades the whole body, (2) the rational part, and also (3) *entrecheia*. * With *entrecheia* we have nothing to do at present, but we have with the other two meanings of soul,

1. The definition must have been something like this: "A πάθος is a διάθεσις resulting from strength or weakness in one of the components of a κρᾶσις." Cf. V. 14–21. A κρᾶσις usually meant in medical language a *perfect* blend of the elements composing a thing. Here it seems to mean a blended mixture, with (possibly) excess or deficiency in the components. Cornford refers to *Phaedo*, 86 b, c, and *Symposium*, 188 a, where κρᾶσις and ἁρμονία are synonyms, so that ἐπίτασις and ἄνεσις (tension and slackness) strictly applicable to the latter can be applied to either.

6. κομίζω in this sense is not noticed by L. and S.

7. For the difficult word δύναμις, see p. 9. Here, perhaps, "vital, or corporeal, or psychic essence".

12. For examples of κινήματα see I. 31. πάθη is used here for the more generic διαθέσεις because abnormal διαθέσεις furnish the best illustrations. The explanation of terms in I. 1–24 is repeated with slight variations in I. 27–II. 19, even the threefold explanation of ψυχή being given twice. Perhaps the student took down the lecturer's revision (or repetition) as well as his original note. For the probable nature of the *Anonymus* papyrus see p. 2.

24. ἐντρέχεια is the best the student could make of the lecturer's ἐντελέχεια.

I καὶ μᾶλλον τοῦ λογιστικοῦ. περὶ γὰρ τοῦτο τὰ προηγούμενα πάθη συνίσ-
ταται καὶ τὰ κατ᾽ ἐπακολούθημα. * πάθη δέ ἐστιν
30 τάδε προηγούμενα κατὰ κείνησιν·
δεισιδαιμονία, λύπη, φόβος, φιλαργυρία·
ταῦτα γὰρ ἐν κεινήσει· * κάρος δὲ καὶ
λήθαργος ἐν σχέσει. * * σωματικὰ δὲ
πυρετός — προηγούμενον μὲν πάθος ἐστὶν
35 τοῦ σώματος, κατ᾽ ἐπακολούθημα δὲ
τῆς ψυχῆς —, μανία ὁμοίως· καὶ ταῦτα ἐν κινήσει τὰ πάθη. * * ἐν σχέσει
δὲ παράλυσις, κάρος, τὰ παραπλήσια·
οὕτω μὲν δὴ χρηστέον τῶι ὅρωι ἐπὶ
40 ἁπάντων. * τῶν δὲ παθῶν τὰ μὲν ψυχικά, τὰ δὲ σωματικά. χρὴ δὲ εἰδέναι
ὅτι τὰ μὲν σωματικὰ πάθη ἀ.....
.......να καὶ περὶ τὴν ζωτικὴν
.......ασται. ὡς ὁμοίως δὲ....

II .. περι...... τοῖς σώμασιν, ὥστε
.. ἰδίας.....άσθαι ταῦτα τήν τε
ζωτικὴν καὶ τὴν ἐν τοῖς σώμασιν
οὖσαν ψυχικήν. ψυχικὸν δ᾽ εἶναι πάθος τὸ
5 τοιοῦτο· διάθεσιν ψυχῆς κατὰ κείνησιν ἢ σχέσιν· καὶ γὰρ ἡ ψυχὴ δύναμίς ἐστιν.
λέγεται δὲ ψυχὴ τριχῶς· ἥ τε ὅλη
καὶ τὸ μέρος τὸ λογιστικὸν καὶ αὐτὴ ἡ

---

36. Perhaps the colon should be after μανία, not ὁμοίως.
I. 42.–II. 4. The sense according to D. is: ἀπὸ τοῦ προηγούμενα καὶ
περὶ τὴν ζωτικὴν δύναμιν εἶναι κατωνόμασται· ὡς ὁμοίως δὲ ψυχικὰ τὰ
περὶ ψυχὴν ὑπάρχοντα τοῖς σώμασιν, ὥστε δυνάμεις ἰδίας κατωνομάσθαι
ταῦτα τήν τε ζωτικήν κ.τ.λ. An alternative would be to take περί with
accusative as part of the phrase περί τι συνίστασθαι occurring in I. 27–29,
which might suggest:

> ὅτι τὰ μὲν σωματικὰ πάθη ἀ⟨εὶ προ-
> ηγούμε⟩να καὶ περὶ τὴν ζωτικὴν
> ⟨δύ⟨ναμιν⟩ συνίστ⟩αται. ὡς ὁμοίως δὲ ⟨τὰ ψυχι-
> κὰ⟩ περὶ ⟨ψυχὴν τὴν ἐν⟩ τοῖς σώμασιν, ὥστε
> ⟨δυ⟨νάμεις⟩⟩ ἰδίας ⟨συνίστ⟩ασθαι ταῦτα, τήν τε
> ζωτικήν κ.τ.λ.

Perhaps ταύτας for ταῦτα (l. 2).

I especially with the rational part. For in this arise both primary affections and also the secondary. * The primary kinetic affections are the following: superstition, pain, fear, avarice. For these are kinetic, * but torpor and coma are static. * Bodily affections are fever—it is a primary affection of the body, as an affection of the soul it is secondary—similarly madness. These affections are kinetic. * In the static class are paralysis, torpor and so on. In this way we must make use of the definition in all cases. *

Of affections some are of the soul, others are of the body. † We must understand that the bodily affections have been so named from their being primary, and concerned with the power of living. Similarly II "psychic" are those affections which arise in the body but concern the soul, so that these have been named special powers, namely the power of living and the psychic power that is in the body; † also that a psychic affection is of the following sort—a condition of the soul either kinetic or static. For in fact the soul is a power. The word "soul" is used in three senses: (1) the whole soul, (2) the rational part and (3) the *entrecheia* itself. But let us deal now with the two former meanings.

28, 29. "Primary" means here "antecedent" and "secondary" is "consequential". προηγούμενον αἴτιον is sometimes used in the sense of a "predisposing" cause.

36. It is extremely odd to say that μανία can "likewise" be a σωματικὸν πάθος, especially as in the Hippocratic *Epidemics* it is used of delirium, which is a typical ψυχικὸν πάθος consequential on the σωματικὸν πάθος of fever. Professor Cornford makes a suggestion which occurred to me independently, namely that Diels has punctuated wrongly. A new sentence should begin at ὁμοίως. "Fever has a consequential affection of the mind, viz. delirium. Similarly, these affections also, as well as those given in ll. 30–32, are kinetic." This is abrupt, but less odd than the punctuation of D.

I. 42–II. 4. The objections to Diels' restoration are (1) its length and (2) the very difficult sense of "bodily affections get their name from their being antecedent and concerned with the power of life". For the sense of my restoration see the analysis of this introductory section, p. 12.

II. 2. ἰδίας, "special", "peculiar", because these are fundamental, basic powers. See p. 13.

6. How can soul be a "power"? Perhaps because it is a sort of "power" (almost Aristotle's ἐντελέχεια) of a living, conscious organism. Contrast, however, I. 19–21.

II   ἐντρέχεια. ἀλλ' ἐπὶ ἐκεῖνα ἴωμεν νῦν· ὅταν γὰρ
10   λέγωμεν συνίστασθαι κατὰ τὴν ψυχὴν
πάθη, περὶ τὴν ὅλην λέγομεν καὶ περὶ
τὸ μέρος αὐτῆς τὸ λογιστικόν. * τῶν τε
ψυχικῶν παθῶν ἃ μέν ἐστιν κατὰ φύσιν, ἃ δὲ
παρὰ φύσιν. παρὰ φύσιν μὲν διαθετικὸν
15   ψυχῆς κατὰ κείνησιν ἢ σχέσιν παρὰ
φύσιν, κατὰ φύσιν δὲ διαθετικὸν ψυχῆς κατὰ κείνησιν ἢ σχέσιν κατὰ φύσιν.
αὕτη μὲν ἡ τεχνολογία τῶν ἀρχαίων ἐστίν,
οἷς καὶ ἡμεῖς ἑπόμεθα. κατα... ουσιν γὰρ
20   καὶ μετριοπαθείας περὶ τὸν σοφόν. καί φασιν
τὰς μετριοπαθείας νεῦρα εἶναι τῶν πρά-
ξεων. οἱ δὲ νεώτεροι, τοῦτ' ἔστιν οἱ Στωικοί,
κατὰ φύσιν πάθος οὐδὲν καταλείπουσιν
ψυχῆς. ταύτηι γάρ φασιν ἐνφέρεσθαι τὸ
25   παρὰ φύσιν ἐκ τῆς πάθους φωνῆς· ἧι
καὶ τὸ πάθος ἀπέδοσαν· πάθος ἐστὶν
ὁρμὴ πλεονάζουσα, τῆς ὁρμῆς αὐτοῖς
ἐξακουομένης οὐχὶ ἀντὶ τῆς ὑπερ-
τάσεως, ἀλλὰ ἀντὶ τοῦ ἀπειθὲς εἶναι τῶι αἱ-
30   ροῦντι λόγωι. ἀλλὰ τοῦτο τοῖς νεωτέροις μελήσει.
ἡμῖν δὲ λεκτέον κατὰ φύσιν πάθη περὶ
τὴν ψυχὴν μνήμην, διαλογισμόν,
τὰ ὅμοια. * παρὰ φύσιν δὲ ἀμνημοσύ-
νην, ἀλογίαν, τὰ ἐοικότα. * * τῶν τε
35   παθῶν τῶν περὶ τὴν ψυχὴν δύο ἐστὶν τὰ
γενικώτατα κατὰ τοὺς ἀρχαίους· ἡδονή τε γὰρ καὶ ὄχλησις, τὰ δὲ μεταξὺ κατ' ἐπίμειξιν γίνεται τῶν εἰρημένων.

---

26 ff. Arius Didymus apud Stob. Ecl. eth. II. 7, 10: πάθος δ' εἶναί
φασιν (Stoici) ὁρμὴν πλεονάζουσαν καὶ ἀπειθῆ τῷ αἱροῦντι λόγῳ ἢ κίνησιν
ψυχῆς ἄλογον παρὰ φύσιν.

---

19. A suitable word would be καταλείπουσιν. Cf. l. 23.
34. Perhaps ἀλογιστίαν.

II For when we say that affections arise in the soul, we are speaking of the whole soul, and also of its rational part. * Of psychic affections some are according to nature and others are contrary to nature. Contrary to nature is an affection which produces a condition of soul, either kinetic or static, that is contrary to nature; according to nature is an affection producing a condition of soul, either kinetic or static, according to nature. This terminology is that of the ancients, whose followers we too are. For "moderate affections" are among the things that they allow to the wise man. They also assert that moderate affections are the sinews of actions. But the younger school, that is to say the Stoics, allow as according to nature no affection of the soul. For into the term, they say, is introduced contrariety to nature from the word "an affection", in virtue of their definition of affection, namely "impulse in excess", impulse being understood by them not in the sense of over-straining, but in the sense of a refusal to listen to the reason that convicts it. But the point must be left to the younger school. We, however, must call memory, reasoning and so on, affections of the soul according to nature; * and contrary to nature forgetfulness, irrationality and the like. * * Of affections of the soul two, according to the ancients, are the most generic—pleasure and distress, and the intermediate affections arise from a combination of those mentioned.

18. Who are the ἀρχαῖοι, so carefully distinguished by Anonymus from the Stoics? He says that in his definition of πάθος he adopts the sense of κρᾶσις that they favoured, which is the sense given to that term by the Cnidian Herodicus (V. 1–21). He also adopts their τεχνολογία of πάθη, adding that they allow μετριοπάθειαι (Peripatetic) to the Sage (II. 12–22). In II. 36 they are said to regard ἡδονή and ὄχλησις (Epicurean) as the most generic of the psychic affections.

It is curious that the treatise *Regimen in Acute Diseases* also speaks of the ἀρχαῖοι, who are there the early Cnidians. These, like the ἀρχαῖοι of *Anonymus* (III. 7–IV. 17), are interested in the nomenclature of diseases and their elaborate subdivision.

We cannot understand by the ἀρχαῖοι "those of old time" generally, because specially distinctive doctrines are attributed to them, marking them out as members of a definite school of thought, though probably only early members are included. In XXIX. 52 and XXX. 17, however, the reference to a particular school is not so clear.

The facts would be covered by the hypothesis that ἀρχαῖοι was an epithet often applied to Cnidians, and that Anonymus used the nomenclature of Aristotelian Epicureans who adopted some of the teaching of Herodicus of Cnidos.

24. ταύτῃ, a μετριοπάθεια, which must be evil if all πάθη are evil.

26, 27. The Stoic definition of πάθος. See *Testimonia*.

29, 30. Cf. ὁ λόγος αἱρεῖ, "the argument proves".

30. The writer seems impatient of philosophical subtleties, this sentence reading like a student's comment on his lecture-notes.

II   κατὰ δὲ τοὺς Στωικοὺς τέσσαρά ἐστιν τὰ
40   γενικώτατα τῆς ψυχῆς πάθη · ἡδονὴ γὰρ καὶ ἐπιθυμία, φόβος τε καὶ λύπη.
καὶ ἡδονὴ μὲν καὶ ἐπιθυμία καθ' ὡς ἂν
ἀγαθοῦ φαντασίαν γίνονται, ὧν ἡ μὲν ἡδονὴ
γίνεται καθ' ὡς ἂν ἀγαθοῦ παρουσίαν, ἐ-
45   φ' ὧι οἷόν τε ἥδεσθαι · εἴδη δὲ αὐτῆς τέρψις, χάρις, τὰ παραπλήσια · ἡ δὲ ἐπιθυμία καθ' ὡς ἂν ἀγαθοῦ γίνεται προσδοκίαν ·
ἐπιθυμοῦμεν γὰρ πάντες προσδοκῶντες

III   τἀγαθόν. * ἥ τε λύπη καὶ ὁ φόβος καθ' ὡς ἂν
κακοῦ φαντασίαν γίνονται, ὧν ὁ μὲν φόβος καθ' ὡς
ἂν κακοῦ προσδοκίαν γίνεται · φοβούμεθα
γὰρ προσδοκῶντες τὸ κακόν. * ἡ δὲ λύ-
5   πη καθ' ὡς ἂν κακοῦ παρουσίαν · λυπού-
μεθα γὰρ ἐπὶ τοῖς παροῦσι κακοῖς. καὶ ταῦτα μὲν οὕτως. * * πάθος δὲ λεκτέον †ειναι σωμα-
τικον† εἶναι σωματικὸν διάθεσιν σώματος
κατὰ κείνησιν ἢ σχέσιν. * * τῶν δὲ σωματι-
10   κῶν παθῶν ἃ μέν ἐστιν τεταγμένα, ἃ δὲ ἄτακτα.
καὶ ἄτακτα μέν ἐστιν πάθη τὰ ἄλλοτε ἄλλως λυόμενα,
οἷον ποτὲ μὲν κατ' ὀλίγον, ποτὲ δὲ ἀθρόως. * τῶν
δὲ τεταγμένων παθῶν ἃ μὲν ἰδίως λέγεται
πάθη, ἃ δὲ νοσήματα. * καὶ ἰδίως πάθη
15   ἐστὶν τεταγμένα τὰ κατ' ὀλίγον λυόμενα.
τῶν δὲ νοσημάτων ἃ μέν ἐστιν ἰδίως νοσήματα,
ἃ δὲ ἀρρωστήματα. καὶ νοσήματα μέν ἐστιν
τὰ ἐμμόνους τὰς κατασκευὰς ἔχοντα
περὶ τὰ σώματα ὑποληπτούς τε χρόνους
20   φερόμενα τῆς λύσεως κατ' ἐλάχιστον.
καὶ γὰρ νοσήματα εἴρηται †αποτου† ἀπὸ τοῦ
ἐννενεοσσευκέναι περὶ τὰ σώματα, ἧι καὶ
διοίσει τὸ τεταγμένον πάθος τοῦ νοσήματος,
καθὸ τὸ μὲν πάθος κατ' ὀλίγον τὴν λύσιν
25   λαμβάνει, τὸ δὲ νόσημα κατ' ἐλάχιστον.

II. 39 ff.   Cf. Arius, l.c.

II. 45.   Perhaps οἴονται.
46.   For χάρις we should probably read χαρά (joy).

II But according to the Stoics the most generic affections of the soul are four in number: pleasure and desire, fear and pain. Pleasure and desire arise with a presentation of what is taken to be a good, and of these pleasure arises with the actual presence of what is taken to be good, at which it is possible to be pleased; its species are delight, gratification and the like. Desire arises with the anticipation of what is taken to be good. For we all desire when we anticipate what is III good. * Pain and fear arise with a presentation of what is taken to be evil. Of these fear arises with an anticipation of what is taken to be evil. * For we fear when we anticipate what is evil. * Pain comes with the presence of what is taken to be evil. For we feel pain when evils are actually present. To pass on. * *

2   We must define a bodily affection as a condition of the body either kinetic or static. * * Of bodily affections some are regular, others irregular. The irregular affections are those that disappear now in one way, now in another; for example, sometimes little by little and at other times all at once. * Of regular affections some are called affections proper, others are lesions. * Regular affections properly so-called are those that disappear little by little. Of lesions some are lesions properly so called, and others are infirmities. Lesions have a permanent constitution in a body, and reach the determinate periods of their disappearance by the least possible stages. In fact lesions are so called because they have "lodged themselves" in a body, wherein too will be the difference between a regular affection and a lesion, in that such an affection disappears little by little, but a lesion by the least

II. 46.   The term χαρά is often associated by the Stoics with τέρψις.
    48.   Or, "anticipate what is good when we desire". Perhaps "expect" would be better than "anticipate".
III. 3, 4.   Or, "anticipate (expect) what is evil when we fear".
    20.   Perhaps "to the least possible degree". Cf. VIII. 41. The writer is more careless than usual in this introductory section of definitions and philosophical terms, taking but little thought to express himself accurately, just as if he considered philosophy out of place in medical lectures. It is indeed difficult, if not impossible, to reconstruct what the lecturer actually said from the garbled notes of his pupil.
    22.   ἐννενεοσσευκέναι. This verb is supposed to be the origin of the word νόσημα. Cf. Plato, Rep. 573 e.
    25.   As in 20 κατ᾽ ἐλάχιστον may mean either (a) "by the least possible stages", as in the translation, or (b) "to the least possible degree", which, while being the normal meaning, seems to fit in less well with the sense of the present passage.

III   τὸ μὲν γὰρ ὀλίγον ἐκ πολλῶν ἐλαχίστων
συνέστηκεν· * τὸ δὲ ἐλάχιστον μέρος
οὐκ ἔχει, ὥστε νόσημα οὐ τεταγμένον.
ἀρρώστημα δὲ τὸ σὺν τῶι κατασκευὴν ἔχειν
30   περὶ τὰ σώματα ἔτι καὶ παρειρῆσθαι τὴν
ῥῶσιν τῶν σωμάτων· ἀπὸ τούτου γὰρ καὶ εἴρηται
ἀρρώστημα. * * διαφέρει δὲ νόσημα
νόσου καὶ ἀρρώστημα ἀρρωστίας. * νόσημα μὲν γάρ ἐστιν ἔμμονος κατασκευὴ περὶ μέρος
35   τι τοῦ σώματος χρόνους ὑπολήπτους
τῆς λύσεως ἔχουσα. * νόσος δὲ ἔμμονος
κατασκευὴ περὶ ὅλον τὸ σῶμα τῆς λύσεως
ὑπολήπτους ἔχουσα χρόνους. * λέγεταί
τε νόσος διχῶς, κοινῶς τε καὶ ἰδίως·
40   κοινῶς μὲν πᾶν παρὰ φύσιν πάθος,
καθ' ὃ σημαινόμενον καὶ ὁ πυρετὸς λέ-
γοιτ' ἂν νόσος. * ἰδίως δὲ ἔμμονος κατασκευὴ περὶ τὰ σώματα τῆς λύσεως ὑπολήπτους ἔχουσα χρόνους. * ἀρ-
45   ρώστημά τε ὡς ὁμοίως λέγεται

IV   κοινῶς τε καὶ ἰδίως· κοινῶς μὲν πάλιν
πᾶν παρὰ φύσιν πάθος, καθ' ὃ σημαινόμενον ὁ πυρεταίνων ἀρρωστεῖν κληθήσε-
ται. * * ἰδίως δὲ κατασκευὴ περὶ τὰ σώματα,
5   ἥτις τῆς λύσεως ὑπολήπτους ἔχει
χρόνους σὺν τῶι παρηρῆσθαι τὴν ῥῶσιν τῶν σωμάτων. * εἰρῆσθαι δὲ τὸ πάθος
συμβέβηκεν ἀπὸ τοῦ παρακολουθοῦντος
ἢ ἀπὸ τόπου. ἀπὸ μὲν γὰρ παρακολουθοῦντος
10   πάθους εἰρῆσθαι τὸν πυρετόν, ἀπὸ τοῦ
πυρῶδ[ε]ς εἶναι τὸ ἐπόμεν[ον καὶ] παράλυσιν
τὸ ἐπόμενον ἐν παραλύσ[ει]· ἀπὸ γὰρ τοῦ λε-
λύσθαι τὸν τόνον. ἀπὸ τόπου δὲ τὴν
ὀνομασίαν ἔσχεν φρενεῖτις· τὸ γὰρ πά-

IV. 14.   Aetius, de plac. IV. 5, 8 (Doxogr. 391 a 20 b, n. 21): οἱ δὲ ἐν τῷ
διαφράγματι scil. τὸ ἡγεμονικὸν τῆς ψυχῆς εἶναι. Caelius Aurelian (i.e.
Soranus), acut. morb. I. 8 (p. 22, ed. Amman, Amst. 1722): aliqui igitur cerebrum
pati dixerunt…alii diaphragma. Soranus in Excerptis Paris. Suppl. cod.
gr. 636, f. 21ᵛ: ὁ δὲ Διοκλῆς φλεγμονὴν τοῦ διαφράγματός φησιν εἶναι
τὴν φρενῖτιν ἀπὸ τόπου καὶ οὐκ ἀπὸ ἐνεργείας τὸ πάθος καλῶν, συνδιατι-
θεμένης καὶ τῆς καρδίας· ἔοικε γὰρ καὶ οὗτος τὴν φρόνησιν περὶ ταύτην
ἀπολείπειν. διὰ αὐτοῦ (scil. διαφράγματος?) γὰρ καὶ τὰς παρακοπὰς
ἕπεσθαι τούτοις.

IV. 11, 12.   Readings doubtful. In l. 10 perhaps πάθος.

III possible stages. For a "little" is composed of many "leasts", * but "the least" has no part, so that a lesion is not regular. An infirmity in addition to its having a constitution in a body is, they say, marked by the body being robbed of its firmness. Hence an infirmity gets its name. * * A lesion differs from a disease and an infirmity from an infirm condition. * For a lesion is a lasting constitution of a part of the body with presumable times for its disappearance; * but a disease is a lasting constitution of the whole of the body with presumable times for its disappearance. * The word "disease" is used in two senses, in a general sense and in a special one. In a general sense every affection contrary to nature is a disease, according to which meaning fever too would be called a disease. * In a special sense it is a lasting constitution of a body with determinate times for its disappearance. * Infirmity too likewise is used in a general sense and a special one. In IV the general sense an infirmity like a disease is any affection contrary to nature, according to which meaning a fever-patient will be called "infirm". * * But in a special sense it is a constitution of the body, which has presumable times for its disappearance, along with the body's being robbed of its firmness. * Affections have come to be named from the attendant affection or from the place affected. For example, a fever is named after the attendant affection, from the fiery nature of the symptom that accompanies it, while in paralysis the accompanying symptom is paralysis, so named from the loss of power to move the sinews. From the place affected *phrenitis* (brain-fever) received its name. For the

III. 28. But see III. 14.

29. ἀρρώστημα is derived by the writer from α privative and ῥῶσις, "strength". The infinitive παρειρῆσθαι is neo-Attic for παρῃρῆσθαι.

IV. 10–13. I.e. *puretos* from *pur*, "fire", and *paralusis* from *para* and *lelusthai*.

14. φρενῖτις was a fever marked by delirium and raving. The seat of intelligence (φρήν, φρένες) was placed by some in the thorax, by others in the brain.

IV 15 θος περὶ τὰς φρένας συνίσταται, οὐχὶ
τὸ διάφραγμα, τοῦτ᾽ ἔστιν τὸ λογιστικὸν μέρος
τῆς ψυχῆς. * * * * * *
.....λο..ος

νόσοι.

20 Περὶ τοῦ προκειμένου δεῖ προλαβεῖν,
ὡς κοινότερον τοῖς ὀνόμασι προσχρώ-
μεθα νόσους ἢ πάθη λέγοντες · τὰς
γὰρ τούτων διαφορὰς γινώσκομέν τε
καὶ ὑπεμνήσαμεν ἐν τοῖς προγεγραμμέ-
25 νοις · * στάσις δὲ περὶ τοῦ ἐκκειμένου.
οἱ μὲν γὰρ εἶπον γίνεσθαι νόσους παρὰ τὰ περισσώματα τὰ γινόμενα ἀπὸ τῆς τροφῆς,
οἱ δὲ παρὰ τὰ στοιχεῖα. καὶ οἱ μὲν ἀρχὴν καὶ ὕλην ὑποθέμενοι τὰ περισσώ-
30 ματα τῶν νόσων λόγους κομίζουσι τοι-
ούτους. * Εὐρυφῶν γάρ τοι ὁ Κνίδιος οἴεται τὰς
νόσους ἀποτελεῖσθαι τρόπωι τοιούτωι ·
ʽὅταν ἡ κοιλία, φησίν, τὴν ληφθεῖσαν
τροφὴν μὴ ἐκπέμπηι, ἀπογεννᾶται
35 περισσώματα, ἃ δὴ ἀνενεχθέντα
ὡς τοὺς κατὰ τὴν κεφαλὴν τόπους
ἀποτελεῖ τὰς νόσους · ὅταν μέντοι γε
λεπτὴ καὶ καθαρὰ ὑπάρχηι ἡ κοιλία, δεόντως
γίνεται ἡ πέψις · ὅταν δὲ μὴ ἦι τοιαύτη,
40 συμβαίνει τὰ προκείμενα γίνεσθαιʼ. * Ἡρόδικος
δὲ ὁ Κνίδιος λέγων περὶ τῆς τῶν νόσων αἰτίας
καὶ αὐτὸς κατὰ μέν τι συναγορεύει

V τῶι Εὐρυφῶντι, κατὰ δέ τι διαφέρει · καθ᾽ ὃ μὲν γὰρ
καὶ αὐτὸς τὰ περισσώματα αἴτια λέγει
τῆς νόσου εἶναι, συμφέρεται · καθ᾽ ὃ δέ φησιν
μὴ διὰ τὸ τὴν κοιλίαν καθαρὰν εἶναι ἢ λεπτήν,
5 διαλλάσσει χρώμενος αἰτίαι τοιαύτηι ·
ὅταν γὰρ ἀκεινητήσαντες οἱ ἄνθρωποι
προσενέγκωνται τροφήν, συμβαίνει
ταύτην μὴ διοικεῖσθαι, ἀλλὰ λιτὴν καὶ

IV. 18.   After thinking that behind the few letters of the papyrus was
concealed some name, D. finally came to the conclusion that we should
read κατὰ πλάτος.

IV affection makes its seat in the *phrenes* (brain, not the diaphragm), which is the rational part of the soul. . . . .

Diseases in detail

3   About this subject it must be first understood that in speaking of diseases and affections we use the words in their more general sense. For the differences between these we know, and have mentioned in what has gone before. * But as to the subject before us there is much difference of opinion. For while some have said that diseases arise because of the residues from nutriment, others hold that they are due to the elements. Those who have postulated the residues as the origin and material of diseases bring forward the following explanations. * Euryphon of Cnidos for example thinks that diseases are caused in the following manner. "When the belly does not discharge the nutriment that has been taken, residues are produced, which then rise to the regions about the head and cause diseases. When however the belly is empty and clean, digestion takes place as it should; otherwise what 4 I have already stated occurs." *

Herodicus of Cnidos, speaking about the cause of diseases, is himself V too partly in agreement with Euryphon, but partly in disagreement. In so far as he himself too says that residues are the causes of disease he is in agreement. In so far as he says that proper digestion is not due to the bowels being clean or empty, he differs, having recourse to the following explanation. When men take in nutriment without previous exercise, the result is that the nutriment is not assimilated, but lying

IV. 18.   For κατὰ πλάτος see Diels' discussion [p. xviii] *Epimetrum*.

25.   περὶ τοῦ ἐκκειμένου is a difficult phrase. Probably τὸ ἐκκείμενον is "the subject before us", and τὸ προκείμενον "the subject already dealt with". Cf. l. 40. The ἐκ- may perhaps call attention to the "lay-out" of the material.

26.   For περίσσωμα see p. 11.

V. 4.   After μὴ understand δεόντως γίνεσθαι τὴν πέψιν. See IV. 38, 39. So D. In classical Greek μὴ would be οὐ (sign of late date).

8.   λιτὴν means literally "plain", "unworked". Here, of course, it means "unaltered".

V
10

ἀκατέργαστον παρακειμένην εἰς περισσώματα ἀναλύεσθαι. * ἐγ μέντοι γε
τῶν περισσωμάτων ἀποτελεῖσθαι δισσὰς ὑγρότητας, μίαν μὲν ὀξεῖαν, τὴν δὲ
ἑτέραν πικράν, καὶ παρὰ τὴν ἑκατέρας
ἐπικράτειαν διάφορα γίνεσθαι τὰ πάθη. λέγει
15 δὲ ὡς παρὰ τὴν τούτων ἐπίτασιν ἢ ἄνεσιν διάφορα ἀπογεννᾶσθαι τὰ πάθη, οἷόν
τι λέγω, ἐὰν ἀνειμένη μᾶλλον ἦι ἡ ὀξεῖα
καὶ μὴ ἄκρατος, ἀναλόγως δὲ καὶ ἡ πικρὰ μὴ ἄγαν ἦι πικρά, ἀλλὰ ἐλασσόνως ἔχηι,
20 ἢ ἐπιτεταμέναι ὦσιν, διάφορα γενήσεσθαι
καὶ τὰ πάθη κατὰ τὰς τῶν ὑγροτήτων κράσεις.
καὶ παρὰ τοὺς τόπους δὲ διάφορα
ἔσται τὰ πάθη· ἐὰν μὲν λόγου εἵνεκα
ἐπὶ κεφαλὴν οἰσθῆι ἡ πικρὰ ὑγρότης,
25 τἀτὸ γενήσεται πάθος, * ἐὰν δὲ
νῦν μὲν ἡ πικρὰ †τηϲ† εἰς τὴν κεφαλὴν
ἐνεχθῆι, νῦν δὲ ἡ ὀξεῖα, γενήσεται
διαλλάσσοντα τὰ πάθη. * ἀλλὰ γὰρ καὶ παρ' αὐτοὺς τοὺς τόπους γενήσεται διαλλάσσοντα
30 τὰ πάθη, ὅταν διάφοροι ὦσιν, ἐφ' οὓς ἡ ἐπιφορά· παρὰ γὰρ τὸ ἐπὶ κεφαλὴν ἢ ἐπὶ ἧπαρ
ἢ σπλῆνα φέρεσθαι τὰς ὑγρότητας
διαφέροντα ἀποτελεσθήσεται τὰ πάθη.
καὶ ἐν τούτοις ἡ τοῦ Ἡροδίκου δόξα.
35 Ἱπποκράτης δέ φησιν αἰτίας εἶναι τῆς νόσου τὰς
φύσας, καθὼς διείληφεν περὶ αὐτοῦ
Ἀριστοτέλης. * ὁ γὰρ Ἱπποκράτης λέγει
τὰς νόσους ἀποτελεῖσθαι κατὰ λόγον
τοιοῦτον· ἢ παρὰ τὸ πλῆθος τῶν

---

39. [Hippocrates], περὶ φυσῶν, 7 (VI. 98, 16 ff. L.): πονηρὴ δέ ἐστιν
ἡ τοιήδε δίαιτα τοῦτο μὲν ὅταν τις πλέονας τροφὰς ὑγρὰς ἢ ξηρὰς διδῶ
τῷ σώματι ἢ τὸ σῶμα δύναται φέρειν καὶ πόνον μηδένα τῷ πλήθει τῶν
τροφῶν ἀντιτιθῇ, τοῦτο δ' ὅταν ποικίλας καὶ ἀνομοίους ἀλλήλησιν ἐσπέμπῃ
τροφάς· τὰ γὰρ ἀνόμοια στασιάζει (cf. VI. 5) καὶ τὰ μὲν θᾶσσον τὰ δὲ
σχολαίτερον πέσσεται. μετὰ δὲ πολλῶν σιτίων ἀνάγκη καὶ πολλὸν πνεῦμα
ἐσιέναι…(VI. 100 L.) ὅταν οὖν τὸ σῶμα πληρωθὲν τροφῆς πλησθῇ καὶ
πνεύματος ἐπὶ πλέον τῶν σιτίων χρονιζομένων (χρονίζεται δὲ τὰ σιτία διὰ
τὸ πλῆθος οὐ δυνάμενα διελθεῖν), ἐμφραχθείσης δὲ τῆς κάτω κοιλίης ἐς
ὅλον τὸ σῶμα διέδραμον αἱ φῦσαι· προσπεσοῦσαι δὲ πρὸς τὰ ἐναιμότατα
τοῦ σώματος ἔψυξαν. τούτων δὲ τῶν τόπων ψυχθέντων ὅπου αἱ ῥίζαι καὶ
αἱ πηγαὶ τοῦ αἵματός εἰσι, διὰ παντὸς τοῦ σώματος φρίκη διῆλθεν· ἅπαντος
δὲ τοῦ αἵματος ψυχθέντος ἅπαν τὸ σῶμα φρίσσει. Ibidem, 8 (VI. 102, 11 L.):
ὁ ἀὴρ ὁ ψύξας τὸ αἷμα κρατηθεὶς (cf. V. 45) ὑπὸ τῆς θερμότητος (cf. περὶ
διαίτης, VI. 520, 13: κρατηθέντος τοῦ ὕδατος).

26.   P. has πικροτης altered to πικρα.

V in the belly undigested and unaltered, it is broken up into residues. *
From the residues however are produced two liquids, one acid, the other
bitter, and the affections turn out different according to the predomi-
nance of one or the other. And he says that according to the strength
or weakness of these the affections resulting are different; what I mean
is, if the acid be on the weak side, and not unblended, and correspondingly if the bitter be not too bitter but on the weaker side, or
if both be strong, the affections also will differ according to the blendings
of the liquids. Affections will be different too according to the
places in which they are found. If for example the bitter fluid be
carried to the head, the same affection will occur, * but if now the
bitter and now the acid fluid be carried to the head, the affections
that result will vary. * But in fact affections will prove variable also
according to the actual places attacked, when these are different. For
affections will turn out different according as the fluids are carried to
head, liver or spleen. Such is the view of Herodicus.

5   But Hippocrates says that breaths (φῦσαι) are causes of disease, as
Aristotle has said in his account of him. * For Hippocrates says that
diseases are brought about in the following fashion. Either be-

18. ἄκρατος, that is, "undiluted", or "without being neutralised".
ἀναλόγως, "correspondingly", i.e. if the bitter be in a condition analogous
to that of the acid in the first example.
35. Scholars have been surprised that to Hippocrates have been attributed
views similar to those of *Breaths*. Dr L. Edelstein thinks that the historical
Hippocrates did hold such views. See Note H. Wellmann believes that
by "Hippocrates" Anonymus means the grandson of the "great"
Hippocrates, who would have been a contemporary of Menon. To us
"Hippocrates" unqualified can refer only to one person, and it is hard
to believe that the name had other associations for Menon, Anonymus or
anyone else.
36. φύσας: perhaps "gases". It is awkward to translate φῦσα and πνεῦμα
by different words, as (at least in the work περὶ φυσῶν) φῦσα *is* πνεῦμα in
the body. See however on XXI. 47.
37. "Aristotle" means Menon's Ἰατρικά composed under the direction
of Aristotle. The language here used shows that the author is paraphrasing
or giving the general sense of the Ἰατρικά, not giving verbally accurate
extracts.

V 40   προσφερομένων ἢ παρὰ τὴν ποικιλίαν
       ἢ παρὰ τὸ ἰσχυρὰ καὶ δυσκατέργαστα εἶναι
       τὰ προσφερόμενα συμβαίνει περισ-
       σώματα ἀπογεννᾶσθαι, καὶ ὅταν
       μὲν πλείονα ἦι τὰ προσενεχθέντα,
45   κατακρατουμένη ἡ ἐνεργοῦσα

VI   τὴν πέψιν θερμότης πρὸς πολλῶν ὄντων
       προσαρμάτων οὐκ ἐνεργεῖ τὴν πέψιν·
       ἀπὸ δὲ τοῦ ταύτην παραποδίζεσθαι
       περισσώματα γίνεται. ὅταν δὲ ποικίλα
5   ἦι τὰ προσενεχθέντα, στασιάζει ἐν τῆι
       κοιλίαι πρὸς ἑαυτά, καὶ κατὰ τὸν στασιασ-
       μὸν μεταβολὴ εἰς περισσώματα. ὅταν
       μέντοι γε ἐλάχιστα καὶ δυσκατέργαστα
       ἦι, οὕτως παραποδισμὸς γίνεται τῆς πέψεως
10   διὰ τὴν δυσκατεργασίαν καὶ οὕτως
       μεταβολὴ εἰς περισσώματα· ἐγ δὲ τῶν
       περισσωμάτων ἀναφέρονται φῦσαι· αἱ δὲ
       ἀνενεχθεῖσαι ἐπιφέρουσι τὰς νόσους. ταῦτα δὲ ἔφησεν ἀνὴρ
       κεινηθεὶς δόγματι τοιούτωι· τὸ γὰρ πνεῦμα
15   ἀναγκαιότατον καὶ κυριώτατον ἀπο-
       λείπει τῶν ἐν ἡμῖν, ἐπειδή γε παρὰ τὴν τού-
       του εὔροιαν ὑγίεια γίνεται, παρὰ δὲ τὴν δύσροιαν
       νόσοι. δίκην τε ἐπέχειν ἡμᾶς φυτῶν·
       ὡς γὰρ ἐκεῖνα προσερρίζωται τῆι γῆι, οὕτως
20   καὶ αὐτοὶ προσερριζώμεθα πρὸς τὸν ἀέρα
       κατά τε τὰς ῥῖνας καὶ κατὰ τὰ ὅλα σώματα.

VI. 14. [Hippocrates], περὶ φυσῶν, 3 (VI. 94, 1 L.): πνεῦμα δὲ τὸ μὲν
ἐν τοῖσι σώμασι φῦσα καλεῖται, τὸ δὲ ἔξω τῶν σωμάτων ὁ ἀήρ. οὗτος δὲ
μέγιστος ἐν τοῖσι πᾶσι τῶν πάντων δυνάστης ἐστίν. Ibidem, 4 (VI. 96, 1):
διότι μὲν οὖν ἐν τοῖς ὅλοις ὁ ἀὴρ ἔρρωται, εἴρηται. τοῖς δ' αὖ θνητοῖσιν
οὗτος αἴτιος τοῦ βίου καὶ τῶν νούσων τοῖσι νοσέουσι. Ibidem, 5 (VI. 96,
13 L.): οὐκ ἄλλοθέν ποθεν εἰκός ἐστι γίνεσθαι τὰς ἀρρωστίας ἢ ἐντεῦθεν,
ὅταν τοῦτο πλέον ἢ ἔλασσον ἢ ἀθρωότερον γένηται ἢ μεμιασμένον
νοσηροῖσι μιάσμασιν ἐς τὸ σῶμα ἐσέλθη.

VI. 8.   Perhaps for ἐλάχιστα should be read πάχιστα.

V cause of the quantity of things taken, or through their diversity, or because the things taken happen to be strong and difficult of digestion, residues are thereby produced, and when the things that have been VI taken are too many, the heat that produces digestion is overpowered by the multitude of foods and does not effect digestion. And because digestion is hindered residues are formed. And when the things that have been taken are of many kinds, they quarrel with one another in the belly, and because of the quarrel there is a change into residues. When however they are very coarse and hard to digest, there occurs hindrance of digestion because they are hard to assimilate, and so a change to residues takes place. From the residues rise gases, which having arisen bring on diseases. What moved Hippocrates to adopt these views was the following conviction. Breath (πνεῦμα), he holds, is the most necessary and the supreme component in us, since health is the result of its free, and disease of its impeded passage. We in fact present a likeness to plants. For as they are rooted in the earth, so we too are rooted in the air by our nostrils and by our whole body. At least we

V. 41. The word ἰσχυρός is particularly common in *Ancient Medicine* to denote the strength or intensity of a "power". We might perhaps compare the language of those people who say that their physician has given them "strong" or "powerful" medicine.

VI. 8. I translate πάχιστα; ἐλάχιστα would be "very few".

13. ἀνήρ is used pronominally for οὗτος.

14. For πνεῦμα see p. 10.

17. See *Breaths*, III, IV and v.

19. What follows is in neither *Breaths* nor any other part of the *Corpus*. Cf. the author's scepticism VI. 42.

VI   ἐοικέναι μέν γε φυτοῖς ἐκείνοις, οἳ στρατιῶται
        καλοῦνται. ὥσπερ γὰρ ἐκεῖνοι προσερρι-
        ζωμένοι τῶι ὑγρῶι μεταφέρονται
25   νῦν μὲν ἐπὶ τοῦτο τὸ ὑγρόν, νῦν δὲ ἐπὶ τοῦ-
        το, οὕτως καὶ αὐτοὶ οἱονεὶ φυτὰ ὄντες
        προσερριζώμεθα πρὸς τὸν ἀέρα καὶ ἐν
        κεινήσει ἐσμὲν μεταχωροῦντες νῦν
        μὲν ἐπὶ τάδε, αὖθις δὲ ἐπ' ἄλλην.
30   εἰ δὲ ταῦτα, φανερὸν ὡς κυριώτατόν ἐστιν
        τὸ πνεῦμα. τούτων ἐκκειμένων, ὅταν γένηται
        περισσώματα, ἀπὸ τούτων γίνονται φῦσαι, αἲ δὴ ἀναθυμιαθεῖσαι
        τὰς νόσους ἀποτελοῦσι· παρά τε τὴν
        διαφορὰν τῶν φυσῶν ἀποτελοῦνται αἱ νόσοι.
35   ἐὰν μὲν γὰρ πολλαὶ ὦσι, νοσάζουσιν,
        ἐὰν δὲ ἐλάχισται, πάλι νόσους ἐπιφέ-
        ρουσι· παρά τε τὴν μεταβολὴν τῶν φυσῶν
        γίνονται αἱ νόσοι· διχῶς δὲ μεταβάλ-
        λουσιν ἢ ἐπὶ τὸ ὑπέρμετρον θερμὸν
40   ἢ ἐπὶ τὸ ὑπέρμετρον ψυχρόν. καὶ ὁποίως ἂν
        γένηται ἡ μεταβολή, νόσους ἀπο-
        τελεῖ. καὶ ὡς μὲν ὁ Ἀριστοτέλης οἴεται
        περὶ Ἱπποκράτους, ταῦτα. * * ὡς δὲ
        αὐτὸς Ἱπποκράτης λέγει, γίνεσθαι τὰς νόσους
45   [παρὰ τὰς διαφορὰς τῶν ἐν τῆι συστά]σει φύσεων

VII   ἀνθρωπ-...................λέ-
        γει δι...........................

VI. 22. Dioscorides, _mater. med._ IV. 100 (I. 593 Spr.): στρατιώτης ὁ ἐπὶ
τῶν ὑδάτων φυόμενος, οἱ δὲ ποτάμιον στρατιώτην καλοῦσιν... ὠνόμασται
δὲ διὰ τὸ ἐπινήχεσθαι τοῖς ὕδασι καὶ χωρὶς ῥίζης ζῆν. φύλλον δὲ ἔχει
ἀειζώου ὅμοιον, μεῖζον μέντοι καὶ ψυκτικὴν ἔχον δύναμιν, ἐφιστάνον τὰς
ἐκ νεφρῶν αἱμορραγίας πινόμενον. τραύματά τε ἀφλέγμαντα τηρεῖ καὶ
ἐρυσιπέλατα καὶ οἰδήματα σὺν ὄξει καταπλασσόμενον ἰᾶται. Pliny, _N.H._
XXIV. 169: celebratur autem et a Graecis stratiotes, sed ea in Aegypto tantum et
inundatione Nili nascitur, aizoo similis ni maiora haberet folia. refrigerat mire
et volnera sanat ex aceto inlita, item ignis sacros et suppurationes. sanguinem
quoque qui defluit a renibus pota cum ture masculo mirifice sistit.

VII. [Hippocrates], περὶ νούσων, I. 2 (VI. 142 L.): αἱ μὲν οὖν νόσοι
γίνονται ἡμῖν ἅπασαι, τῶν μὲν ἐν τῷ σώματι ἐνεόντων, ἀπό τε χολῆς καὶ

VI. 34. P. has φυ altered to νοσοι. D. thinks that διάφοροι may have
fallen out before νόσοι.

VI are, he says, like those plants that are called "soldiers". For just as they, rooted in the moisture, are carried now to this moisture and now to that, even so we also, being as it were plants, are rooted in the air, and are in motion, changing our position now hither now thither. If this be so, it is clear that breath (πνεῦμα) is the supreme component. On this theory, when residues occur, they give rise to breaths, which rising as vapour cause diseases. The variations in the breaths cause the various diseases. If the breaths are violent [many], they produce disease, as they also do if they are very light [few]. The changes too of breaths give rise to diseases. These changes take place in two directions, towards excessive heat or towards excessive cold. The nature of the change determines the character of the disease. This is Aristotle's view of Hippocrates. * *

6 But what Hippocrates himself says is that diseases are caused by the differences in the elemental components of the human organism.............

VII.............

....

VI. 22–25. Dr Charles Singer says that duckweed behaves in this way.

29. ἄλλην: understand χώραν.

31. For ἐκκειμένων see note on IV. 25.

35, 36. It is difficult to decide whether πολλαί and ἐλάχισται refer to quantity or number. The same difficulty occurs in many parts of the Corpus, particularly when the reference is to excreta. I have discussed the matter in my Hippocrates, vol. I. pp. lxi, lxii of the General Introduction.

42. That is, of course, Menon's.

44. See Nature of Man, IV and XV.

45. Doubt has been thrown by Fredrich (in his de libro περὶ φύσιος ἀνθρώπου pseudippocrateo) on this meaning of φύσις in the plural. He thinks it cannot mean "elementary bodies", ἰδέαι. But if φύσις can mean "primal matter", "really existent material", the plural can, logically and grammatically, mean elements. Whether it is idiomatically correct is scarcely to the point, as Anonymus is not careful in his use of philosophical terms, being impatient of all such niceties. See e.g. II. 30.

VII. 1–11. Fredrich has restored a little of the undecipherable portion of this chapter by using the vocabulary and phrases of Diseases I. His restoration, however, gives us very little of the sense other than what we might have guessed from the surviving words of the papyrus itself. On the other hand, it is something to know that some authorities—perhaps Menon himself—looked upon Diseases I as by Hippocrates.

VII   ἢ ὑπ...........................
5   ταῦτα ἐπὶ δὴ γινομένοις..............
     καὶ οὖσι συνίστασθαι..........τοῦ
     παρόντος φλέγματος..............ων
     εἶναι ἐν ἡμῖν κατὰ φύσιν τὸ αἷμα........
     τῶν ἰατρῶν· παρὰ φύσιν τε τὴν εἰς........
10   ὅτι αὗται μὲν ἐν ἡμῖν γίνονται αἱ νόσοι διὰ τῆς
     φλεγμασίας. τάδε γὰρ ἐκτὸς...........
     πόνων ὑπερμέτρων, καταψύξεως, θερμότητος.
     παρά τε τὴν τῆς χολῆς καὶ τοῦ φλέγματος
     κατάψυξιν ἢ θερμότητα περιγίνεσθαι τὰς νό-
15   σους· * * ἀλλὰ γὰρ ἔτι φησὶν Ἱπποκράτης γίνεσθαι τὰς
     νόσους ἢ ἀπὸ τοῦ πνεύματος ἢ ἀπὸ τῶν διαι-
     τημάτων, καὶ τούτων τὴν ὑποτύπωσιν δοκεῖ οὕτως
     ἐκτίθεσθαι· ὅταν μὲν γάρ, φησίν, ὑπὸ τῆς αὐ-
     τῆς νόσου πολλοὶ ἁλίσκωνται ἅμα, τὰς
20   αἰτίας ἀναθέσθαι δεῖ τῶι ἀέρι· παρὰ γὰρ

φλέγματος, τῶν δὲ ἔξωθεν ἀπὸ πόνων καὶ τρωμάτων καὶ ὑπὸ τοῦ θερμοῦ
ὑπερθερμαίνοντος καὶ τοῦ ψυχροῦ ὑπερψύχοντος. καὶ ἡ μὲν χολὴ καὶ
τὸ φλέγμα γινομένοισί τε συγγίνεται καὶ ἔνι ἀεὶ ἐν τῷ σώματι ἢ πλέον
ἢ ἔλασσον· τὰς δὲ νόσους παρέχει τὰς μὲν ἀπὸ σιτίων καὶ ποτῶν, τὰς
δὲ ἀπὸ τοῦ θερμοῦ ὑπερθερμαίνοντος καὶ ἀπὸ τοῦ ψυχροῦ ὑπερψύχοντος.
Ibidem, 24: τὸ δὲ ῥῖγος...ἰσχυρότερον γίνεται, ὅταν χολὴ καὶ φλέγμα
συμμιχθῇ ἐς τὠυτὸ τῷ αἵματι ἢ τὸ ἕτερον ἢ ἀμφότερον· μᾶλλον δὲ ἢν
τὸ φλέγμα συμμιχθῇ· ψυχρότατον γάρ...τὸ φλέγμα, θερμότατον δὲ
αἷμα, ψυχρότερον δὲ καὶ χολὴ τοῦ αἵματος κ.τ.λ. Ibidem, 34: καὶ ψύχεος
δὲ καὶ πυρὸς καὶ πόνων ἀρχὴν ταύτην ἴσχει· ὅταν τὸ αἷμα ἐν τῇσι φλεψὶν
ὑπὸ τοῦ φλέγματος ψυχθῇ, μεταπίπτει...καὶ ἀποθνήσκει.

VII. 16. [Hippocrates], περὶ φύσιος ἀνθρώπου, 9 (VI. 52, 11 L.): αἱ δὲ
νοῦσοι γίνονται αἱ μὲν ἀπὸ τῶν διαιτημάτων αἱ δὲ ἀπὸ τοῦ πνεύματος

5. ἐπειδὴ Wilamowitz.
11. αἵδε δὲ γίγνονται Wilamowitz. D. supplies: τάδε γὰρ ἐκτὸς γίνεσθαι
παρὰ φύσιν ἀπό. Fredrich has tried to reconstruct VII. 1–12 from περὶ
νούσων, I. 24, 34. See his de libro περὶ φύσιος ἀνθρώπου pseudippocrateo,
pp. 28–31. Here are his reconstructions:
2   διὰ πόνους ἢ τραύματα
3   ἢ ὑπερβολὴν ψυχροῦ ἢ θερμοῦ τὰς δὲ ἐντὸς ἀπὸ
4   χολῆς καὶ φλέγματος
5   ταῦτα ἐπὶ δὴ γινομένοις
6   καὶ οὖσι συνίστασθαι
7   παρόντος φλέγματος
8   εἶναι ἐν ἡμῖν κατὰ φύσιν τὸ αἷμα χωρισθέντων
9   τῶν ψυχρῶν, παρὰ φύσιν δὲ τὴν εἰς τὰτὸ μῖξιν.

VII . . . .

. . . .

. . . .

. . . .

that these diseases arise in us through inflammation. For these things apart from . . . . of excessive fatigue, chill or heat. And it is because of the chilling or heating of bile and of phlegm that diseases result. * * But as a matter of fact Hippocrates goes on to say that diseases have their origin in either the air (πνεύματος) or regimen, and the outline of these matters he thinks fit to set out thus. Whenever, he says, many are attacked at one and the same time by the same disease, the cause must be attributed to the air.[1] For if the air produce a disease,

[1] Or "atmosphere".

VII τοῦτον γίνεται ἡ αὐτὴ νόσος. * * ὅταν μέντοι πολλὰ εἴδη καὶ ποικίλα γίνηται νόσων, αἴτια, φησίν, λεκτέον τὰ διαιτήματα, οὐχ ὑγιῶς ποι-
ούμενος τὴν ἐπιχείρησιν. ἐνίοτε γὰρ
25 τὸ αὐτὸ αἴτιον πολλῶν καὶ ποικίλων
νοσημάτων γίνεται· κατασκευαστικὸν γάρ-
τοι πλῆθος καὶ πυρετοῦ καὶ πλευρίτι-
δος καὶ ἐπιληψίας ἐστίν, ὅπερ κατὰ σύστασιν
τῶν σωμάτων ἀναδεχομένων τίκτει
30 καὶ τὰς νόσους. οὐ γὰρ δὴ πάντων σωμάτων,
ἐπεὶ ἕν ἐστιν αἴτιον, ἤδη μία καὶ νόσος φέρεται,
ἀλλ᾽, ὥσπερ εἴπομεν, πολλὰ καὶ ποικίλα εἴδη.
καὶ τἄμπαλιν ἔστιν ὅτε ὑπὸ διαφερόντων αἰτίων
τἀτὰ γίνεται πάθη. καὶ γὰρ διὰ πλῆθος ἡ κοιλία
35 ῥεῖ, ἔτι καὶ διὰ δριμύτητα, εἰ χολὴ παραρρεῖ.
ἐξ ὧν φανερόν, ὡς ψεύδεται περὶ τούτων ἀνήρ,
ὡς προϊόντος ἐπιδείξομεν τοῦ λόγου. * * ἐκεῖνο
μέντοι γε ῥητέον, διότι ἄλλως Ἀριστοτέλης περὶ τοῦ Ἱπποκράτους λέγει καὶ
40 ἄλλως αὐτός φησιν γίνεσθαι τὰς νόσους. * * οἷς ἑπό-
μενος ὁ Ἀβυδηνὸς Ἀλκαμένης
λέγει γίνεσθαι τὰς νόσους, ὥς φησιν περὶ
αὐτοῦ Ἀριστοτέλης, διὰ τὰ περισσώματα τὰ ἀπὸ τῆς τροφῆς κατασκευα-

---

ὃ ἐσαγόμενοι ζῶμεν· τὴν δὲ διάγνωσιν χρὴ ἑκατέρου ὧδε ποιεῖσθαι· ὅταν
μὲν ὑπὸ ἑνὸς νοσήματος πολλοὶ ἄνθρωποι ἁλίσκωνται κατὰ τὸν αὐτὸν
χρόνον, τὴν αἰτίην χρὴ ἀνατιθέναι τούτῳ, ὅτι κοινότατόν ἐστι καὶ μάλιστα
αὐτῷ πάντες χρώμεθα. ἔστι δὲ τοῦτο ὃ ἀναπνέομεν· φανερὸν γὰρ δὴ ὅτι
τὰ διαιτήματα ἑκάστου ἡμῶν οὐκ αἴτιά ἐστιν, ὅτε γε ἅπτεται πάντων ἡ
νοῦσος ἑξῆς καὶ τῶν νεωτέρων καὶ τῶν πρεσβυτέρων καὶ γυναικῶν καὶ
ἀνδρῶν ὁμοίως.

21. Hippocrates, περὶ φύσιος ἀνθρώπου, 9 (54, 6 L.): ὅταν δὲ αἱ
νοῦσοι γίνωνται παντοδαπαὶ κατὰ τοὺς αὐτοὺς χρόνους, δῆλον ὅτι τὰ
διαιτήματά ἐστιν αἴτια ἕκαστα ἑκάστοισι, καὶ τὴν θεραπείην χρὴ ποιεῖσθαι
ἐναντιούμενον τῇ προφάσει τῆς νούσου, ὥσπερ μοι πέφρασται καὶ ἑτέρωθι,
καὶ ἐκ τῶν διαιτημάτων μεταβάλλειν. Ibidem (54, 17 L.): ὅταν δὲ νοσήματος ἑνὸς ἐπιδημίη καθεστήκῃ καὶ δῆλον ᾖ, ὅτι οὐ τὰ διαιτήματα αἴτιά
ἐστιν, ἀλλ᾽ ὃ ἀναπνέομεν τοῦτ᾽ αἴτιόν ἐστι, δῆλον ὅτι τοῦτο νοσηρὴν τὴν
ἀπόκρισιν ἔχον ἂν εἴη. τοῦτον χρὴ τὸν χρόνον τὰς παραινέσιας ποιεῖσθαι
τοῖσιν ἀνθρώποισιν τοιάσδε· τὰ μὲν διαιτήματα μὴ μεταβάλλειν, ὅτι γε
οὐκ αἴτιά ἐστι τῆς νούσου, τὸ δὲ σῶμα ὁρᾶν, ὅπως ἔσται ἀογκότατον κτλ.

VII it will be the same one. * * When, however, many different forms of diseases occur, we must attribute them to errors of regimen, he says, employing an unsound method of argument. For there are times when many different diseases have one and the same cause. For surely fever, pleurisy and epilepsy may be the result of a surfeit, which produces diseases corresponding to the constitution of the body that takes it in. For certainly one and the same cause does not bring one and the same disease to every body, but, as we have said, many and various forms. On the other hand, sometimes different causes produce the same affection. For diarrhœa is caused through surfeit, as well as through acridness if there be any untoward flow of bile. From these facts it is manifest that Hippocrates is mistaken in this matter, as we

7 shall show in the course of our narrative. * * Yet it must be said that what Aristotle tells us about him does not tally with Hippocrates' own statements about the origin of diseases. * *

Following whom Alcamenes of Abydos, according to the account of him given by Aristotle, says that diseases occur through the residues

37. ἀποδείξομεν: the promise is not fulfilled.

VIII

ζόμενα· αἴτια γὰρ ταῦτα τῶν νόσων εἶναι. κατὰ
τοῦτο μέντοι γε διάφορος φαίνεται π-
ρὸς τὸν Εὐρυφῶντα, καθ' ὅσον κατά τι
μὲν [τ]ὴν κεφαλὴν εἶπεν ἐπι[κου]-
5 ρικὴν γίνεσθαι τῶν περιττωμάτων, ἁπλῶς
δὲ ὁ Ἀλκαμένης εἶπεν· " ἀνατρέχοντα
μὲν ὡς τὴν κεφαλὴν τὰ περισσώματα γίνεται ἐπιχορηγούμενα πρὸς τῆς κεφαλῆς καὶ ἐπιπεμπόμενα τῶι ὅλωι
10 σώματι τὰς νόσους ἐμποιεῖ." * * ὁ δὲ
Μεταποντῖνος Τιμόθεος, καθώς
φησιν περὶ αὐτοῦ ὁ αὐτὸς φιλόσοφος,
λέγει ἀποτελεῖσθαι τὰς νόσους τρόπωι τούτωι· ὅταν μὲν γὰρ ἡ κεφαλὴ ὑγιὴς
15 ἦι καὶ †καθαρα† καθαρά, καὶ ἡ τροφὴ ἀπ' αὐτῆς προστίθεται τῶι ὅλωι σώματι †και ο†
ὑγιαίνει τὸ ζῶιον· * ὅταν δὲ μὴ ὑγιὴς
ἦι, νόσους ἐπιφέρει τῶι τὰς διεξόδους
ἀποφράσσεσθαι· " ὅταν γάρ, φησίν, αὗται ἀποφρα-
20 γῶσιν, ἀνατρέχον τὸ περίσσωμα
ὡς τοὺς κατὰ τὴν κεφαλὴν τόπους
τέως τῶι μὴ ἔχειν διέξοδον ἐν-
μένει, ἐνμεῖναν δὲ μεταβάλλει
εἰς ἁλμυρὸν καὶ δριμὺ ὑγρόν, καὶ εἶτα
25 πλείονα ἐνμεῖναν χρόνον καὶ ῥῆξιν
ἐργασάμενον φέρεται εἰς ὁτιοῦν μέρος.
καὶ παρὰ τὰς τούτου διαφορὰς διαφόρους
τὰς νόσους ἐπιφέρει. * ἔστι δ' ὅτε, φησίν, καὶ
ἀθρόως οἰσθὲν ἐπὶ τὴν τραχεῖαν
30 ἀρτηρίαν — λάρυγξ δὲ αὕτη — πνιγμοὺς
ἐπιφέρει καὶ συντόμους ἐξαγωγὰς
.....νην." * νοσεῖν δέ φησιν τὴν κεφαλὴν ἢ δι' ὑπερβολὴν καταψύξεως ἢ δι' ὑπερβολὴν θερμότητος ἢ διὰ πληγήν. * *

---

16. We must either retain καὶ or change προστίθεται to προστί-
θηται.
32. D. suggests κατὰ ἀγχόνην.

VIII arising from nutriment, these residues being the causes of disease.

He appears, however, to be at variance with Euryphon in that Euryphon restricted the aid given by the head to the residues; but Alcamenes said simply: "The residues rushing up to the head are reinforced by the head, and being disseminated throughout the whole body produce diseases in it." * *

8 But Timotheus of Metapontum, according to the statements about him made by the same philosopher, says that diseases are brought about in the following manner: whenever the head (?) is healthy and clean, the nutriment is added from it to the whole body, and the creature is healthy; * but whenever the head (?) is not healthy, then it brings on diseases by the passages being blocked. "For when", he says, "these are blocked, the residue mounts to the parts about the head, and for a while remains there because it has no passage, but, after remaining, changes to salt and acrid moisture, and then after remaining for a longer time it forces a breach and is carried to some part or other of the body. The position of the part determines the character of the particular disease caused. * Sometimes, he says, it is carried all together to the windpipe, that is the larynx, producing chokings and short gasps. * The head, he says, may be diseased through excess of chill or through excess of heat or through a blow. * *

5. ἁπλῶς: "without qualification", "roundly", "bluntly", "without troubling about exceptions or details"—a difficult word to translate adequately without clumsy paraphrase.

12. "The same philosopher", i.e. "Aristotle", or rather, Menon.

14. The papyrus has clearly κεφαλή, but D. says "lege κοιλία". Surely a mere slip on the part of a weary medical student, and not ignorance, as D. rather unkindly suggests: "caput et ventrem confundere (VIII. 14) non cuiusvis est", p. xv.

32. The suggested κατὰ ἀγχόνην is literally "by strangling".

VIII 35 Ἄ.ας δὲ ἰδίως οἴεται γίνεσθαι τὰς νόσους
διὰ τὰς τοῦ ἐνκεφάλου καθάρσεις.
καθαίρεσθαι δὲ τὸν ἐγκέφαλον διὰ
μυκτήρων, ὤτων, ὀφθαλμῶν,
στόματος, κατά τε τὰς διαφορὰς τοῦ πλήθους τῶν κα-
40 θάρσεων ὑγίειαν γίνεσθαι ἢ νόσον. ὅταν μὲν γὰρ
κατ' ἐλάχιστον γένηται ἡ κάθαρσις,
ὑγιαίνει τὸ ζῷον, * ὅταν δὲ ὑπερ-
κόρως, νοσεῖ. λέγει δὲ διὰ ταύτας
τὰς καθάρσεις γίνεσθαι πέντε κατάρρους

About two lines are missing.

...ιτωι μη....................
κατάρρους. * *...................
5 Ἡρακλεόδωρος....................
.. ενομεν......................
τὴν αὐτὴν.....................
. δύο εἶπον.....................
...ς παρα......................
10 .. εν ὅταν.....................
τὸ σῶμα ὑγιαίνει (?).................

VIII. 35. [Hippocrates], περὶ τόπων τῶν κατ' ἄνθρωπον, I (VI.276, 12 L.):
ἡ γὰρ κοιλίη ὁπόταν ὑπεκχώρησιν μὴ ποιῇ τὴν μετρίην καὶ ἐσιῇ ἐς αὐτήν,
ἄρδει τῇ ὑγρότητι τὸ σῶμα τῇ ἀπὸ τῶν σιτίων τῶν προσφερομένων· αὕτη
δὲ ἡ ὑγρότης ἀπὸ τῆς κοιλίης ἀποφρασσομένη ἐς τὴν κεφαλὴν ὡδοιπόρησεν
ἀθρόη, καὶ ἐς τὴν κεφαλὴν ἐπὴν ἀφίκηται οὐ χωρευμένη ὑπὸ τῶν τευχέων
τῶν ἐν τῇ κεφαλῇ, ῥεῖ ᾗ ἂν τύχῃ καὶ πέριξ τῆς κεφαλῆς καὶ ἐς τὸν
ἐγκέφαλον διὰ λεπτοῦ τοῦ ὀστέου...καὶ ἢν μὲν ἐς τὴν κοιλίην πάλιν
ἀφίκηται, τῇ κοιλίῃ νοῦσον ἐποίησεν, ἢν δ' ἄλλη πῃ τύχῃ, ἄλλη νοῦσον
ποιεῖ.
44. [Hippocrates], περὶ τόπων τῶν κατ' ἄνθρωπον, 10 (VI. 294, I L.): ῥόοι
δὲ ἀπὸ τῆς κεφαλῆς ἑπτά· ὁ μὲν κατὰ τὰς ῥῖνας ὁ δὲ κατὰ τὰ ὦτα ὁ
δὲ κατὰ τοὺς ὀφθαλμούς. οὗτοι οἱ ῥόοι καταφανέες ἐκ τῆς κεφαλῆς τοῖσιν
ὀφθαλμοῖσιν. ἐπὴν δ' ἐς τὸν κίθαρον ῥυῇ ὑπὸ ψύχους, χολὴ γίνεται...
ὅταν δ' ἐς τὸν μύελον ῥόος γένηται, φθίσις ἀλαῖα γίνεται. ὅταν δ' ὄπισθεν
ἐς τοὺς σπονδύλους καὶ ἐς τὰς σάρκας ῥυῇ, ὕδρωψ γίνεται...(296, 6) ἢν
δ' ὀλίγον ῥεύσῃ, ἰσχιάδα καὶ κέδματα ἐποίησεν. [Hippocrates], περὶ ἀδένων,
11 (VIII. 564, 18 L.): ῥόοι δὲ ἀπὸ κεφαλῆς ἕως ἀποκρίσιος δι' ὤτων κατὰ
φύσιν, δι' ὀφθαλμῶν, διὰ ῥινῶν· τρεῖς οὗτοι· καὶ ἄλλοι δι' ὑπερῴης ἐς
φάρυγγα, ἐς στόμαχον, ἄλλοι διὰ φλεβῶν ἐπὶ νωτιαῖον, ἐς τὸ αἷμα [τὰ
ἰσχία L.], οἱ πάντες ἑπτά.

VIII. 35. For δὲ ἰδίως K. suggests δ' ὁ Ἰασεύς.

VIII. 9   But Aias is peculiar in thinking that diseases are caused through the

purgings of the brain.   The brain is purged, he says, by way of nostrils,

ears, eyes and mouth, and according to the variations in the amount of

the purgings is produced health or disease.   For when the cleansing is at

a minimum, the creature is in health, * but when in excess it is diseased.

IX And he says that through these purgings five catarrhs occur . . . .

10 . . . .

VIII. 35.   The name may be Abas, but no physician is known of either
name.
44.   See *Testimonia.*
IX. 1–19.   In this big gap occurs the name Heracleodorus, an unknown.

IX   τως νόσοι........................

   ται τὰ σώματα...................

   ρα προσενεχθέντα (?)...............

15   πλήθη, ἀλλὰ αἷσπερ..............

   καὶ τὰς νόσους.................δυσ-

   κρότως ἐχ.....................

   μετρίαν νόσον...................

   καὶ κατάψυξιν...................

20 Ἡρόδικος δὲ ὁ Σηλυμβριανὸς οἴεται
   τὰς νόσους γίνεσθαι ἀπὸ τῆς διαίτης· ταύτην δὲ εἶναι κατὰ φύσιν, ὅταν πόνοι προσῶσιν
   καὶ ἄλγη δ᾽ ὅσα δεῖ, καὶ οὕτως πέψιν μὲν
   ἔχῃ ἡ τροφή, ἐπίδοσιν δὲ ἀεὶ λαμβάνῃ
25 τὰ σώματα ἀναδιδομένης τῆς τροφῆς κατὰ
   φύσιν. οἴεται γὰρ τὴν μὲν ὑγίειαν γίνεσθαι κατὰ
   φύσιν ἐχόντων τῶν σωμάτων περὶ τὴν δίαιταν, τὴν δὲ
   νόσον παρὰ φύσιν ἐχόντων αὐτῶν. τοῖς μέντοι
   παρὰ φύσιν διατεθεῖσιν πονεῖν προστάσσει
30 ἡ ἰατρικὴ παραγομένη καὶ οὕτως εἰς τὸ κατὰ
   φύσιν ἄγει ταῦτα, ὡς αὐτός φησιν. * λέγουσιν
   δὲ τὸν ἄνδρα τὴν ἰατρικὴν ἔντεχνον
   ἀγωγὴν εἰς τὸ κατὰ φύσιν καλέσαι. * καὶ ταῦτα μὲν
   οὕτως, ἐκεῖνο δὲ ὅτι ἀπ᾽ ἐναντίων τῆς τε
35 θερμότητος καὶ ὑγρότητος τῶν σωμάτων
   συνίστανται νόσοι, διατεθρύληται. * *

---

20. [Hippocrates], *Epidem.* VI. 3, 18 (V. 302 L.): Ἡρόδικος τοὺς
πυρεταίνοντας ἔκτεινε δρόμοισι, πάλῃσι πολλῇσι, πυρίῃσι. κακόν. τό
πυρετῶδες πολέμιον πάλῃσι, περίοδοι δρόμοισιν, ἀνατρίψει. πόνος πόνῳ.
Galen (XVII. B 99 K.): καὶ Πλάτων μὲν μέμνηται τοῦ Ἡροδίκου ὡς πολλοῖς
περιπάτοις χρωμένου. τίνος γε νῦν Ἡροδίκου μνημονεύει [Hippocrates],
πότερον τοῦ Λεοντίνου ἢ τοῦ Σηλυμβριανοῦ περιττὸν ζητεῖν. Plato, *Rep.* III.
406 a–c; *Prot.* 316 d; *Phaedr.* 227 d: ἔγωγ᾽ οὖν οὕτως ἐπιτεθύμηκα ἀκοῦσαι,
ὥστ᾽ ἐὰν βαδίζων ποιῇ τὸν περίπατον Μεγαράδε, καὶ κατὰ Ἡρόδικον
προσβὰς τῷ τείχει πάλιν ἀπίῃς, οὐ μή σου ἀπολειφθῶ. Aristotle, *Rhet.*
A 5, 1361 b 4: πολλοὶ γὰρ ὑγιαίνουσιν ὥσπερ Ἡρόδικος λέγεται, οὓς οὐδεὶς
ἂν εὐδαιμονίσειε τῆς ὑγιείας διὰ τὸ πάντων ἀπέχεσθαι τῶν ἀνθρωπίνων ἢ
τῶν πλείστων. Cf. Pliny, *N.H.* XXIX. 4.

22. Cf. [Hippocrates], *περὶ φυσῶν,* 7 (VI. 98 L.): πονηρὴ δέ ἐστιν ἡ
τοιήδε δίαιτα τοῦτο μὲν ὅταν τις πλέονας τροφὰς ἢ ὑγρὰς ἢ ξηρὰς διδῷ
τῷ σώματι ἢ τὸ σῶμα δύναται φέρειν καὶ πόνον μηδένα τῷ πλήθει τῶν
τροφῶν ἀντιτιθῇ.

36. Perhaps αἱ should be supplied before νόσοι.

IX . . . .

. . . .

. . . .

. . . .

11 But Herodicus of Selymbria thinks that diseases come from regimen.

Regimen, he says, is according to nature when it includes exercise, and the proper amount of discomfort too, so that the nourishment is digested, and the body continually receives its increase, as the nourishment is absorbed according to nature. For he thinks that health results when the body enjoys a natural regimen, and disease when the regimen is unnatural. Those, however, who are in an unnatural condition medicine, when called in, bids take exercise, and so, as he himself says, brings them to the natural condition. * It is said too that this writer called the art of medicine "scientific guidance to the natural condition". * In addition to these opinions there is a popular view that diseases result from the conflict of two opposites—heat and moisture—in our bodies. * *

20. For the ancient authorities for Herodicus see *Testimonia*.
22. "Natural" or "normal".
35. The theme of [Hippocrates], *Regimen*, I–IV. All that has been said about Herodicus fits in with the argument of this book, so that it is quite possible that he, or rather a pupil (because of dates), was its author. Possibly διατεθρύληται may mean "is constantly reiterated" (in *Regimen*).

IX   ὁ δὲ Αἰγύπτιος Νινύας ἰδίως λέγει τὰ μὲν
      συγγενικὰ γίνεσθαι πάθη, τὰ δὲ ἀλλότρια *
      καὶ τὰ μὲν συγγενικὰ ἔμφυτα τοῖς σώμασιν
40   εἶναι. * ὑπὸ δὲ ἄλλης αἰτίας συνίστασθαι
      τὰς νόσους τρόπωι τοιούτωι· ὅταν γὰρ
      ἡ τροφὴ ληφθεῖσα μὴ ἀναδοθῆι τῶι σώματι,
      ἀλλ᾽ ἐνμείνηι, ἡ θερμότης ἡ ἐν ἡμῖν οὖσα περισσώματα
      ἐξ αὐτῆς ἀπογεννᾶι...............

                About twenty-six lines missing

X 27 ....ινος
      ....νόσους
      ....μὲν εἶναι
30   ....επι.ν
      ....μιον
      ....αμα
      ....ενον
      ....απαρα
35   ....μὴ διὰ
      ....ἀλγηδόν
      ....μενος
      ....
      ....δύναμιν
40   ....ε
      ....ιον
      ....σκευ-
      ....αμεν δὲ
      ....ψυχ..

                About six lines missing

XI 7 ....ν καὶ ὑγίειαν
      ....ἀλμυρὰν δὲ
      ....εμενος..
10   .... * καὶ....
      ....φις
      ....τοὺς νεφροὺς
      ....τὴν θερμὴν
      ....ιον μέγα
15   ....ἡ δὲ πυρρὰ
      ....καὶ πρασο-

IX. 12   Ninyas the Egyptian is peculiar in dividing affections into congenital

and acquired, * the congenital, he says, being innate in our bodies. *

He holds that there is another cause, by which diseases are produced

in the following way. Whenever nutriment is taken that is not absorbed

into the body, but remains in the organs, the warmth in us generates

out of this nutriment residues.

X . . . .

XI

    IX. 37.   Ninyas is an unknown.

XI εἰδῆς.............ατος τὸ αἷμα
    ....αίτατον
    ....μα το....ον ἡ δὲ μέλαι-
20 να........ντων....μένων ὑποστάσε-
    ων........αἷμα....τόπον ἔχει
    ......ε...ς * * Ἵππων δὲ ὁ Κροτω-
    νιάτης οἴεται ἐν ἡμῖν οἰκείαν εἶναι ὑγρότη-
    τα, καθ᾽ ἣν καὶ αἰσθανόμεθα καὶ †υγιαι
25 νομεν† ᾗ ζῶμεν· ὅταν μὲν οὖν οἰκείως ἔχηι
    ἡ τοιαύτη ὑγρότης, ὑγιαίνει τὸ ζῷον,
    ὅταν δὲ ἀναξηρανθῆι, ἀναισθητεῖ τε
    τὸ ζῷον καὶ ἀποθνήσκει. διὰ δὴ τοῦτο
    οἱ γέροντες ξηροὶ καὶ ἀναίσθητοι, ὅτι
30 χωρὶς ὑγρότητος· ἀναλόγως δὴ τὰ πέλ-
    ματα ἀναίσθητα, ὅτι ἄμοιρα ὑγρότητος.
    καὶ ταῦτα μὲν ἄχρι τούτου φησίν. * ἐν ἄλλωι
    δὲ βυβλίωι αὐτὸς ἀνὴρ λέγει τὴν κα-
    τωνομασμένην ὑγρότητα μεταβάλ-
35 λειν δι᾽ ὑπερβολὴν θερμότητος καὶ
    δι᾽ ὑπερβολὴν ψυχρότητος καὶ οὕτως νόσους
    ἐπιφέρειν. * μεταβάλλειν δέ φησιν αὐτὴν
    ἢ ἐπὶ τὸ πλεῖον ὑγρὸν ἢ ἐπὶ τὸ ξηρό-
    τερον ἢ ἐπὶ τὸ παχυμερέστερον
40 ἢ ἐπὶ τὸ λεπτομερέστερον ἢ εἰς ἕτερα. καὶ τὸ αἴτιον οὕτως
    νοσολογεῖ,
    τὰς δὲ νόσους τὰς γινομένας
    οὐχ ὑπαγορεύει. * * Θρασύμαχος
    δὲ ὁ Σαρδιανὸς αἰτίαν ἀπολείπει τῶν νόσων
    τὸ αἷμα· κατὰ δὲ τὴν τούτου μεταβολὴν

XII ἀποτελεῖσθαι τὰς νόσους. μεταβάλλειν δὲ ἢ δι᾽ ὑπερβολὴν
    καταψύξεως ἢ δι᾽ ὑπερβολὴν θερμότη-
    τος. * τὴν δὲ μεταβολὴν τοῦ αἵματος γίνεσθαι
    ἢ εἰς φλέγμα ἢ χολὴν ἢ σεσηπός. * καὶ
5   τὸ μὲν αἷμα ἁπλοῦν, τὴν δὲ χολὴν καὶ
    τὸ φλέγμα καὶ τὸ σεσηπὸς ποικίλα

XI. The first part deals with the various kinds of bile.
22. The name Ἵππων is doubtful, but "doctrina quidem est Hipponi unice apta" (D.).
XII. 2. καταψυχεως P.

XI. 13   But Hippon of Croton believes that there is in us a natural moisture

whereby we perceive and by which we live. Now when such moisture

is in its normal condition, the animal is healthy, but when it dries up,

the animal loses consciousness and dies. This is the very reason why

old men are dry and lack feeling—they are without moisture. Similarly

the soles of the feet, lacking moisture, have no feeling. Hippon pursues

the subject no further, * but in another book the same writer says

that the above-mentioned moisture changes through excess of heat

and excess of cold, and so brings on diseases. * It changes, he says, in

the direction of greater moistness, or of greater dryness, of greater

coarseness, of greater fineness, or into other substances. In this manner

he accounts for disease, but he does not indicate the diseases that result

from the various causes. * *

14   But Thrasymachus of Sardis makes blood the cause of diseases, the

XII changes of blood producing each its disease. The changes of blood

occur, he says, through excess of cold or through excess of heat, *

blood changing into 'phlegm, or bile, or pus; * blood is simple; but

XI. 22.   Hippon was a belated Ionian who revived the teaching of Thales.
42.   Thrasymachus is another unknown.

XII ὄντα ποικίλας καὶ διαφόρους ἐπιφέρειν
νόσους. * * πάντα δὲ ὁμοίως φησὶν Δέξιππος ὁ Κῷος, ὃς οἴεται συνίστασθαι τὰς νόσους
10 ἀπὸ τῶν τῆς τροφῆς περιττωμάτων,
τοῦτ' ἔστιν ἀπό τε χολῆς καὶ φλέγματος δυνάμεων γινομένων
περὶ μέρος καὶ περὶ ὅλον,
κεινουμένων τούτων μὴ ἐξ ἑαυτῶν, ἀλλὰ
παρὰ τὰς πολλὰς καὶ ἀκαίρους τῆς τροφῆς δόσεις.
νοσοποιεῖν δὲ ταῦτα καὶ παρὰ τὸ πλῆ-
15 θος καὶ παρὰ τὸν τόπον καὶ εἶδος, μεταβάλλειν δὲ οἴεται καὶ δι' ὑπερβολὴν
πάντων· καὶ γὰρ θερμότητος καὶ ψύξεως
ἢ τοιούτων παραπλησίων· καὶ περὶ μὲν
τούτου φαίνεται παραπλησίως τοῖς
20 πρότερον αἰτιολογῶν. * περιττό-
†το†τερος δὲ αὐτῶν φαίνεται κατὰ τοῦτο·
λέγει γὰρ τηκομένης τῆς χολῆς καὶ
τοῦ φλέγματος καὶ ὑγροτέρων γινομένων
ἀποτελεῖσθαι ἰχῶρας καὶ ἱδρῶτας·
25 σηπομένων δὲ αὐτῶν καὶ παχυνομένων
ἐπιφέρειν ἦχον, μύξας, λήμας· ἀνα-
ξηράνσει δὲ στερεῶν ἀποτελεσθέντων
πιμελὴν καὶ σάρκας γίνεσθαι ἐξ αὐτῶν
λέγει............καὶ αἷμα
30 π..............λεγόμενα
χολήν......φλέγματος ἐπιμειχθέντος
τῶι αἵματι ...μα ...τὸ φλέγμα
.......νθέντος δὲ αὐτοῦ λευκὸν
φλέγμα γίνεται, μελανθέντος δὲ καὶ μετα-
35 βληθέντος μέλαινα χολή. καὶ ἡ μὲν
τοῦ Κώιου δόξα τοιαύτη. * * Φασίλας
δὲ ὁ Τενέδιος λέγει συνίστασθαι
τὰς νόσους ἢ παρὰ τὴν ἀποφορὰν
τῶν ἐν ἡμῖν ὑγροτήτων καὶ προστι-
40 θεμένων ἀνοικείοις τόποις ἢ ἀπὸ τῶν
ἀποχωρημάτων αὐτῶν· εἶναι γάρ φησιν ἐν ἡμῖν
κατὰ φύσιν ὑγρότητας καὶ τὰς μὲν
†τὰς† ὑγρότητας οὐ κατονομάζει

8. Perhaps πάντα δὲ ὁμοίως, φησίν (scil. Menon), Δέξιππος ὁ Κῷος
οἴεται.
28. Restored by H. Schöne.
36. φασιλας or φασιτας P.

XII bile, phlegm and pus, being of various sorts, bring on diseases too

that are various and different. *

Entirely similar are the views of Dexippus the Coan, who thinks

15 that diseases are produced from residues of nutriment, that is from the

powers of bile and phlegm arising in a part of the body or in the whole,

these being stirred up, not of themselves, but through many unseason-

able partakings of nutriment. These things cause disease, he says, by

reason of their quantity, position and form, and he considers that

change takes place also through excess of anything—of heat, of cold, or

of similar things. In this he plainly accounts for disease in a way similar

to the thinkers mentioned above, * but he appears to elaborate their

view in stating that bile and phlegm melt, and as they become more

liquid, sera and sweats are produced. These thicken and become pus,

resulting in noise in the ears, mucus and rheum. When by drying there

have been produced solids, there arise from them, he says, fat and the

various forms of flesh.....................................

........phlegm being mixed with the blood,......when it has

lost all its colour there arises white phlegm, and when it has changed

and blackened, black bile. Such are the views of the Coan physician. * *

16 But Phasilas of Tenedos says that diseases are caused either by the

emanation from the moistures in us, that become attached to unsuitable

places, or from the excretions themselves. For he says that there are in

us natural moistures, and while to the moistures he does not give names

yet...

8. Dexippus: see p. 14.
11. For the difficult word δύναμις see p. 9
36. Phasilas is another unknown.

XIII τ........................
o........................
αἷμα......................
κατὰ τά..................
5 ἀποχώρημα..................
τόπ.......................
η.........................
ται ἢ ὅταν................
ἅπασαι. *.................
10 φησὶ συνίστασθαι τὰς νόσους ἐκ τοῦ
φλέγματος.................,.
λαμβάνει..................
ἐξ ἑαυτῶν· εἰ δὲ ἐπὶ................
αὕτη γὰρ ἐπιμείνασα............. ται διατιθεισῶν τὸ ὅλον
σῶμα
15 λέγει ηγετοι ..τόποισ....
προειρημένα μὴ καθ᾽ ἑαυτά, μετὰ δὲ
καὶ τῆς τοῦ σώματος διαθέσεως· ωσ.ε
ἐὰν γὰρ ἔχηι ὑπὸ νόσου τὸ ζῷον ηελ....ν
εὐκρότως μὲν γὰρ αὐτοῦ διακειμένου
20 ὑγίεια γίνεται, δυσκρότως δὲ νόσος.
Αἰγίμιος δὲ ὁ Ἠλεῖος οἴεται γίνεσθαι τὰς νόσους
ἢ διὰ πλῆθος τῶν περισσωμάτων ἢ διὰ τροφήν.
γινόμενον δὲ τὸ πλῆθος.. †καιτ νοσοποιεῖν
μὴ ἅπαξ, ἀλλὰ καὶ πλεονάκις. * συνίστασθαι
25 δέ φησιν τὸ πλῆθος τῶν περισσωμάτων τρόπωι
τοιούτωι· * σύντηξις γίνεται ἀπὸ τῶν σωμάτων, ἥτις ἀποκρίνεται τῆι μὲν κατὰ τὸ λόγωι
θεωρητόν, τῆι δὲ καὶ κατὰ τὸ αἰσθητόν, —
διὰ δὲ κοιλίας, οὔρων, ὤτων, μυκτήρων,
30 στόματος —, τῶν ἄλλων ἀποκρίσεων γινομένων
κατὰ λόγον. εἰ μὴ γὰρ αὖ σύντηξις ἐγίνετο
ἀπὸ τῶν σωμάτων, εἰς ἄπειρον ἂν μετ᾽ ὀλίγον
αὔξετο τὰ ἡμέτερα σώματα· * καὶ δεόν-
τως· προσθέσεως γὰρ γινομένης,
35 μηκέτι δὲ ἀποφορᾶς, εὔλογον ἦν αὔξησιν
γίνεσθαι ἐπὶ πλεῖον. * ἐπεὶ δὲ οὐ μόνον πρόσθεσις
γίνεται τοῖς σώμασιν, ἀλλὰ πρὸς λόγον τῆς προσθέ-

18. The sense apparently is ἢ ζῇ ἢ ἀποθνήσκει.

XIII ....

....

17 he says that diseases are caused by the phlegm...............

....

....

already mentioned not by themselves, but with the condition also of

the body. For according to the effect of disease upon it the creature

lives or dies. For when it is in a state of harmony health results, when

harmony is bad, disease.

18 Aegimius of Elis holds that diseases occur either through the bulk

of the residues or through nutriment. When the bulk has collected * *

causes disease, he says, not once but often. * The bulk of residues is

produced, he says, in the following way. * Colliquescence takes place

from our bodies, the fluid being secreted as we can partly infer,

partly perceive, through the belly, the urine, the ears, the nostrils

and the mouth, the other secretions taking place in a corresponding

manner. For if on the other hand colliquescence did not take place

from bodies, our bodies would grow after a while to a vast size, *

and so it must be. For if addition took place while nothing were

taken away, growth would naturally go on and on. * But since

not only do our bodies increase but also, through the before-

21. For Aegimius see p. 14.   24. For μὴ see p. 33.

26. What is the relation of σύντηξις to περισσώματα? Apparently
σύντηξις is the resolution of non-assimilated food into liquid form, which
either is evacuated or roams about the body. See p. 11.

30. What are "the other secretions"? Perhaps the meaning is: "secretions generally follow this rule".

XIII   σεως καὶ ἀποφορὰ διὰ τῶν κατωνομασ-
       μένων ἀποκρίσεων, ταύτηι ἐπ' ἐλάχιστον
40   ἢ αὔξησις τῶν σωμάτων. * * φησὶν δὲ τρέφεσθαι
       τὰ σώματα ὑπὸ τῆς νεαρᾶς καὶ ἀπέ-
       πτου τροφῆς, γενηθείσης δὲ τῆς πέ-
       ψεως καὶ ἀναδόσεως κενοῦσθαι τὰ
       ἀγγεῖα καὶ τὰς διεξόδους. * * τὸ δὲ
45   πλῆθος συνίστασθαι εἰσφερομένης
       ἑτέρας τροφῆς, πρὶν τὴν πρώτην
       πέψεως τυχεῖν. * * ὅταν γὰρ πρότερον

XIV   ... τὴν τροφὴν π ....
       ....
       καὶ ὅσοι μὲν οὖν τὰς νόσους γίνεσθαι λέγουσιν
       διὰ τὸ πλῆθος, μάλιστα ἀπὸ τῶν
5   περισσωμάτων αἰτιολογοῦντες,
       σχεδὸν εἴρηνται. * * ἴδωμεν δὲ καὶ
       τοὺς ἀπὸ τῶν περισσωμάτων καὶ
       διακρίσεων αἰτιολογοῦντας τὰς
       νόσους καὶ τοὺς ἀπὸ τῆς τῶν στοιχείων
10   συστάσεως οἰομένους συνεστάναι τὰ
       ἡμέτερα σώματα. καὶ πρῶτον ἀπὸ
       Πλάτωνος. οὗτος γάρ φησιν τὰ ἡμέ-
       τερα σώματα συνίστασθαι ἐκ τῶν
       τεσσάρων στοιχείων, ὅτι καὶ τὰ ἐν κόσ-
15   μωι [γίνεται] ἀνὰ λόγον. διαφέρειν δὲ ταῦτα·

XIV. 14.   Plato, *Timaeus*, 31 b–32 c. Cf. Aristotle, *de gen. et inter.* A 10,
328 a 5 : ἐπεὶ δ' οὐκ ἔστιν εἰς τἀλάχιστα διαιρεθῆναι, οὔτε σύνθεσις ταὐτὸ καὶ
μίξις ἀλλ' ἕτερον δῆλον ὡς οὔτε κατὰ μικρὰ σῳζόμενα δεῖ τὰ μιγνύμενα
φάναι μεμῖχθαι. σύνθεσις γὰρ ἔσται καὶ οὐ κρᾶσις οὐδὲ μῖξις, οὐδ' ἕξει τὸν
αὐτὸν λόγον τῷ ὅλῳ τὸ μόριον. φαμὲν δ' εἴπερ δεῖ μεμῖχθαί τι τὸ μιχθὲν
ὁμοιομερὲς εἶναι καὶ ὥσπερ τοῦ ὕδατος τὸ μέρος ὕδωρ, οὕτω καὶ τοῦ κρα-
θέντος. ἂν δ' ᾖ κατὰ μικρὰ σύνθεσις ἡ μῖξις, οὐθὲν συμβήσεται τούτων, ἀλλὰ
μόνον μεμιγμένα πρὸς τὴν αἴσθησιν. Arius Didymus apud Stob. *Ecl. eth.*
I. 17 (463, 20 *Doxogr.*): διαφέρειν γὰρ ἀρέσκει τοῖς ἀπὸ τῆς Στωικῆς αἱρέσεως
παράθεσιν, μῖξιν, κρᾶσιν, σύγχυσιν. παράθεσιν μὲν γὰρ εἶναι σωμάτων
συναφὴν κατὰ τὰς ἐπιφανείας, ὡς ἐπὶ τῶν σωρῶν ὁρῶμεν, ἐν οἷς πυροί τε
καὶ κριθαὶ καὶ φακοὶ καὶ εἴ τινα τούτοις ἄλλα παραπλήσια περιέχεται
καὶ τῶν ἐπὶ τῶν αἰγιαλῶν ψήφων καὶ ἄμμων. μῖξιν δ' εἶναι δύο ἢ καὶ

XIV. 6.   Some suggest μετὰ for καὶ.
15.   For γίνεται K. suggests doubtfully τέσσαρα.

XIII mentioned secretions, decrease proportionally to the increase, the

growth of our bodies is reduced to a minimum. * * And he states

that our bodies are nourished by fresh and undigested nutriment, but

when digestion and absorption have taken place the vessels and the

passages are emptied. * * The surfeit collects when other nutriment

is introduced before the first is digested. * * For when before . . . . . the

XIV nutriment * * digestion . . . .

19 Those who state that diseases are caused by surfeit, accounting for

them mainly by residues, have been practically all mentioned. * * After

those who attribute the causes of diseases to residues and secretions, let

us take a glance at those too who hold that our bodies are composed of

a combination of the elements. Let us begin with Plato. He says that

our bodies are composed of the four elements, because the things too

in the world come into being through a proportional compounding.

XIV. 6. I translate μετὰ for καί.

15. The phrase ἀνὰ λόγον is curious. The reference is to *Timaeus*
31 b–32 c, where Plato discusses the ἀναλογία of the elements of the cosmos.
"The god set water and air between fire and earth, and made them, so far
as was possible, proportional to one another, so that as fire is to air, so is
air to water, and as air is to water, so is water to earth." Cornford, *Plato's
Cosmology*, p. 44.

XIV σύνφθαρσιν, μῖξιν, διάκρασιν. * καὶ σύνφθαρσιν μὲν καὶ σύγχυσιν, ὅταν σώματα
διὰ ἑαυτῶν ὅλων ἥκοντα μίαν ὑπεράνω
ἀποτελέσηι ποιότητα, ὡς ἐπὶ τῆς τετρα-
20 φαρμάκου. * μῖξις δέ ἐστιν, ὅταν σώματά τινα ἑαυτοῖς κατὰ παράθεσιν παρακέηται
καὶ μὴ δι᾽ ἑαυτῶν ἥκηι, ὡς σωρὸς πυροῦ,
κριθῆς. * διάκρασις δέ ἐστιν, †οταν† ὅταν σώματά
τινα ἐπὶ ἓν συνελθόντα ἀλλήλοις
25 παρακέηται, ὡς ἐπὶ τοῦ οἰνομέλιτος
βλέπομεν. ἀπὸ τοιγάρτοι τῆς τούτων διαφορᾶς
φησιν ὁ Πλάτων τὰ ἡμέτερα σώματα
ἐκ τῶν τεσσάρων στοιχείων συνεστάναι
κατὰ σύνφθαρσιν. ταύτηι δὲ μὴ φαίνεσθαι καθ᾽ ἓν
30 ἐν ἡμῖν πῦρ ἢ ἀέρα ἢ γῆν ἢ ὑγρὸν τῶι
κατὰ σύνφθαρσιν αὐτῶν τὰ ζῶια ἀποτελεῖσθαι * * ἀλλὰ γὰρ λέγει ἀνὴρ καί
τινα τῶν ἐν ἡμῖν μερῶν διαφόρου τε-
τευχέναι κράσεως ἐκ τῶν στοιχείων.

πλειόνων σωμάτων ἀντιπαρέκτασιν δι᾽ ὅλων, ὑπομενουσῶν τῶν συμφυῶν
περὶ αὐτὰ ποιοτήτων, ὡς ἐπὶ τοῦ πυρὸς ἔχει καὶ τοῦ πεπυρακτωμένου
σιδήρου· ἐπὶ τούτων γὰρ δι᾽ ὅλων γίγνεσθαι τῶν σωμάτων τὴν ἀντιπαρέκτασιν. ὁμοίως δὲ κἀπὶ τῶν ἐν ἡμῖν ψυχῶν ἔχειν. δι᾽ ὅλων γὰρ τῶν
σωμάτων ἡμῶν ἀντιπαρεκτείνουσιν· ἀρέσκει γὰρ αὐτοῖς σῶμα διὰ σώματος
ἀντιπαρήκειν. κρᾶσιν δὲ εἶναι λέγουσι δύο ἢ καὶ πλειόνων σωμάτων ὑγρῶν
δι᾽ ὅλων ἀντιπαρέκτασιν τῶν περὶ αὐτὰ ποιοτήτων ὑπομενουσῶν. [τὴν
μὲν μῖξιν καὶ ἐπὶ ξηρῶν γίγνεσθαι σωμάτων, οἷον πυρὸς καὶ σιδήρου
ψυχῆς τε καὶ τοῦ περιέχοντος αὐτὴν σώματος· τὴν δὲ κρᾶσιν ἐπὶ μόνων
φασὶ γίνεσθαι τῶν ὑγρῶν.] συνεκφαίνεσθαι γὰρ ἐκ τῆς κράσεως τὴν
ἑκάστου τῶν συγκραθέντων ὑγρῶν ποιότητα οἷον οἴνου, μέλιτος, ὕδατος,
ὄξους, τῶν παραπλησίων. ὅτι δ᾽ ἐπὶ τοιούτων κράσεων διαμένουσιν αἱ
ποιότητες τῶν συγκραθέντων πρόδηλον ἐκ τοῦ πολλάκις ἐξ ἐπιμηχανήσεως
ἀποχωρίζεσθαι ταῦτα ἀπ᾽ ἀλλήλων. ἐὰν γοῦν σπόγγον ἠλαιωμένον καθῆ
τις εἰς οἶνον ὕδατι κεκραμένον, ἀποχωρίσει τὸ ὕδωρ τοῦ οἴνου ἀναδραμόντος
τοῦ ὕδατος εἰς τὸν σπόγγον. τὴν δὲ σύγχυσιν δύο ἢ καὶ πλειόνων ποιοτήτων
περὶ τὰ σώματα μεταβολὴν εἰς ἑτέρας διαφερούσης τούτων ποιότητος
γένεσιν, ὡς ἐπὶ τῆς συνθέσεως ἔχει τῶν μύρων καὶ τῶν ἰατρικῶν φαρμάκων. Philo, de aetern. mundi, 16, p. 503 M. 25, 23 Cumont: κατὰ δὲ
σύγχυσιν ὡς ἡ παρὰ ἰατροῖς τετραφάρμακος.
26. Plato, Tim. 82a.

29. K. thinks P. has σύνθεσιν or σύγκρασιν.
32. τελεῖσθαι K.

XIV We must distinguish the following: blending, mixing, compounding. *

We have blending or fusion when bodies interpenetrate throughout, and result in one supervening quality, as in the case of the tetrapharmacos. * It is mixing when bodies lie by each other in juxtaposition, and do not pervade each other, as in the case of a heap of wheat or barley. * It is compounding when bodies lie by each other after combining into one, as we see in the case of "wine-and-honey". Accordingly, on the basis of the difference between these processes Plato says that our bodies are composed out of the four elements by blending. Thus there is not manifest in us, he holds, fire singly, or air, or earth, or moisture, because it is by a blending of them that animals are formed. * * As a matter of fact this authority states also that certain of our limbs have a combination of the elements different from that of others. For the head is not

16–32.   Attributed to Plato, but really Stoic doctrine. See the quotation in the *Testimonia* from Stobaeus. A sheer mistake on the part of either lecturer or student.

19, 20.   The τετραφάρμακος was a compound of wax, tallow, pitch and resin. It was used as a plaster for promoting suppuration: Celsus v, 19, 9.

25.   οἰνόμελι was a kind of mead—a mixture of wine and honey.

29.   The negative in classical Greek would have been οὐ.

XIV 35 οὐ γὰρ ὡσαύτως κέκραται κεφαλὴ
ἢ χείρ, ἀλλὰ ἄλλως μὲν κεφαλή, ἄλλως
δὲ θώραξ, ἐπεὶ κοινῶς ἕκαστον τῶν
ἡμετέρων σωμάτων διαφόρου κράσεως
τετύχηκεν, ὅθεν καὶ αὐτὰ διάφορα ἑαυτῶν. * ἔτι γε μήν φησιν
ὡς ὁ μυελὸς
40 συνέστηκεν ἐκ τῶν τεσσάρων στοιχείων καὶ κύριος εὐθύς ἐστι τῶν ἐν ἡμῖν
ἁπάντων, χρώμενος πιθανότητι λόγων
τοιαύτηι· ἀνῆφθαι γὰρ ἐκ τοῦ μυελοῦ
τὴν ψυχὴν τὴν τὸ ὅλον σῶμα διοικοῦσαν

XV   Three lines illegible
κυριώτατ-......................
5 καὶ μὴν τ......................
καὶ.......................
ὑστ........................
καὶ ἀνι.......................
χοις .να......................
10 καὶ ἅμα......................
δ.ν τοῖς......................
.....το......................
....
ἀεὶ τὰ βόεια...................
15 λέγει δευτερ-..................
χει....αι....................
στοιχείων ἐχ...................
συνεστηκ......................
κοιλ†ε†ιῶν κα..................
20 ἐκκειμένων. * διαιρῶν δὲ τὸν μυελὸν εἰς
μέρη τινὰ κατὰ ἕκαστον μέρος διάφορον σχῆμα ἀποδίδωσιν· τὸ γὰρ ἐνκεφάλου σχῆμα λεγόμενόν φησιν εἶναι καὶ περιφερὲς καὶ κεκυκλωμένον, * τοῦ δὲ λοι-
25 ποῦ μυελοῦ ὁ νωτιαῖος περιέχουσι

XIV. 39. Plato, *Tim.* 73a–74a.
XV. 14 (?). Plato, *Rep.* I. 338c.

XIV. 41. Perhaps P. has κυριως or κυριωτατος (in contraction).

XIV a combination like that of the hand, but the head has a different combination, and the chest yet another, since in general each part of our bodies possesses an individual combination different from that of others, which accounts for their individual differences. * Moreover, he says that the marrow is composed of the four elements, and is directly master of all things that are in us, relying on the plausibility of the following argument. The soul, he affirms, which pervades the whole body, has been attached to the marrow..

XV ....And dividing the marrow into certain parts, he assigns to the several parts different shapes. For what we call the brain (the "head-enclosed") he says is both round and enclosed in a globe. * and of the other marrow the spinal is assigned

XIV. 37. With ἔκαστον must be understood μέρος. This is grammatically very awkward, as σῶμα would be the natural complement. This is another instance of the linguistic carelessness of Anonymus.

XV. 22–24. "Das sogenannte Gehirn, sagt er, habe eine runde und kugelige Form." B. and S. "The brain's shape, so called, he says is both circular and rounded", i.e. circular with a dome.

This seems to be the obvious meaning of the reading of P. But the words of Plato, Timaeus, 73 c, d, καὶ τὴν μὲν τὸ θεῖον σπέρμα οἷον ἄρουραν μέλλουσαν ἕξειν ἐν αὐτῇ περιφερῆ πανταχῇ πλάσας ἐπωνόμασε....ἐγκέφαλον, seem to suggest (1) that περιφερὲς is not "circular" but "spherical", and (2) that λεγόμενον refers to the literal meaning of ἐγκέφαλον, "in the head" (ἐν κεφαλῇ). But if so, what is κεκυκλωμένον? In 44 d Plato says: τὸ τοῦ παντὸς σχῆμα ἀπομιμησάμενοι περιφερὲς ὄν, εἰς σφαιροειδὲς σῶμα ἐνέδησαν, τοῦτο ὃ νῦν κεφαλὴν ἐπονομάζομεν. This points to the meaning "enclosed in a sphere" for κεκυκλωμένον. "The shape of the 'head-contained', as we style the brain, he says is both spherical and enclosed in a globe", i.e. the head. Logically λεγομένου would be more correct, and this perhaps should be read.

XV ὀστέοις καταλείπεται στέγειν. αὐτῆς †τε
τηϲ† τε τῆς ψυχῆς ȳ μέρη εἶναι λέγων
τὸ μὲν λογιστικὸν [ὡς ὀχυρωτάτωι] τῶι ἐνκε-
φάλωι ἀπολείπει, τὸ μέντοι ἄλογον μέρος
30 αὐτῆς ἐν τῶι νωτιαίωι μυελῶι. συνεστάναι δέ φησιν τὰ ὀστέα μίξει γῆς τε καθαρᾶς
καὶ μυελοῦ, ἐναλ[λαγῆναι δὲ τ]οῦ πυρός
τε αὐτὰ ἐνπήξει [καὶ τετηκότος. * * τὴν]
δὲ σάρκα συνεστάναι ἔκ τε γῆς καὶ ὕδατος
35 καὶ πυρὸς καὶ ζύμης τινὸς ἐχούσης ὑ-
γρότητα ἁλμυράν τε καὶ δρειμεῖαν. * * παρεσ-
πάρθαι δ᾽ ἐν τῆι σαρκὶ καὶ ὑγροτέραν τινὰ
θερμότητα πεποιημένην. * τὸ ὑγρὸν
δὲ ἐν ταῖς ὑπερβαλλούσαις ἐνκαύσεσι
40 τη†ι†κόμενον ψύχειν τὴν θερμασίαν, ἐν
ταῖς δὲ ὑπερβαλλούσαις ψύξεσιν ἐναν-
τιοῦσθαι καὶ θερμὸν παρέχεσθαι τὸ
σῶμα. * τὰς δὲ πλείστας σάρκας εἶναι
περὶ τὰ ἀψυχότερα τῶν ὀστῶν· περὶ μηροὺς
45 γὰρ καὶ κνήμας καὶ γλουτοὺς πολλὰς
σάρκας ὑπάρχειν, ἐπειδήπερ αὐτῶν τὰ
ὀστέα ἀψυχότερά ἐστιν, * * περὶ δὲ τὴν κεφα-

XVI λὴν ὀλίγας, * περὶ [δὲ γλῶσσαν ποιεῖ]ται αὐτῆς
ὀστέα τἀψυχότερα μεστά. * ἀμέλει ἀρ-
γεῖν φησιν τὰ παχέα· λέγεσθαι γάρ· "παχεῖα γαστὴρ

XV. 26. Plato, Tim. 69 d–e.
31. Plato, Tim. 80 e–81 c.
33. Plato, Tim. 74 c–d: ταῦτα ἡμῶν διανοηθεὶς ὁ κηροπλάστης, ὕδατι
μὲν καὶ πυρὶ καὶ γῇ ξυμμίξας καὶ ξυναρμόσας, ἐξ ὀξέος καὶ ἁλμυροῦ
ξυνθεὶς ζύμωμα ὑπομίξας αὐτοῖς σάρκα ἔγχυμον καὶ μαλακὴν ξυνέστησε.
36. Plato, Tim. 74 b–c.
43. Plato, Tim. 74 e–75 a.
XVI. 1. Plato, Tim. 75 a–c.
3. Cf. Galen, v. 878 K.: καὶ τοῦτο πρὸς ἁπάντων σχεδὸν ἀνθρώπων
ᾄδεται, διότι πάντων ἐστὶν ἀληθέστατον, ὡς γαστὴρ ἡ παχεῖα τὸν νοῦν οὐ
τίκτει τὸν λεπτόν.

XV. 26. στέγειν (restored from Tim. 73 d στέγασμα) is doubtful.
33. Perhaps τοῦ ὕδατος for καὶ τετηκότος. The article is not wanted,
but may perhaps be generic, as in "hardened in the fire".
XVI. 2. τἀψυχοτερα P.: τὰ ψυχρότερα K.

XV to the protection of the bones that surround it. Of the soul itself he says that there are three parts, placing in the brain, as being very strong, the rational part, but its irrational part in the spinal marrow. Bones, he says, are composed by mixing pure earth and marrow, and hardened by alternate use of fire and melted (?). * * Flesh is composed of earth, water, fire and a sort of leaven with a salt and acrid moisture. * * Dispersed in flesh is also a moister sort of warmth that has been created. * The moisture in excessive heats getting thinner cools the heat, and in excessive cold opposes it and makes the body warm. * Most of the flesh is around such bones as have less life in them. For around thighs, shins, and buttocks there lies abundance of flesh, since in their bones is

XVI less of life. * * Around the head, however, is but little flesh, * but full of it are the more lifeless bones that grow around the tongue. * Of course, he says, gross things do no work, as the proverb puts it, "A gross

XV. 33. I suspect that the text is corrupt. My proposed emendation ("solidified by alternate use of fire and water") is strongly supported by *Tim.* 73e: τὸ δὲ ὀστοῦν...καὶ μετὰ τοῦτο εἰς πῦρ αὐτὸ ἐντίθησι, μετ᾽ ἐκεῖνο δὲ εἰς ὕδωρ βάπτει, πάλιν δὲ εἰς πῦρ αὖθίς τε εἰς ὕδωρ. Perhaps the lecturer was not heard clearly by the note-taker. Cornford suggests ἐναλλαγῇ δ᾽ ὑγροῦ πυρός τε or ἐναλλὰξ δ᾽ ὑφ᾽ ὑγροῦ, adopting my idea that ἄτηκτα should be read for ἐνπήξει, but can make nothing of καὶ τετηκότος.
37. Or, "a warmth that has been made rather moist".
XVI. In this chapter the original is paraphrased with some freedom.
3. A verse quoted *inter alios* by Gregorius Naz. ΙΙ. p. 213 d.

XVI λεπτὸν οὐ τίκτει νόον." * * τά τε ὀστέα φησὶν
5 πεπηγέναι ἀποστηρίγματος χάριν.
ἄρθρα δὲ αὐτοῖς πεποιῆσθαι πρὸς τὰς συ-
στολὰς καὶ κάμψεις. * νεῦρα δὲ τούτοις
ἔξωθεν .. τὴν σκληρότητα τῶν ὀστῶν
διὰ τὰς κατὰ προαίρεσιν κεινήσεις. * σάρκας
10 δὲ διὰ προβολὴν ψύχους τε καὶ θάλπους. * τά τε νεῦρα συνεστάναι ἐξ
σαρκὸς ἀζύμου καὶ ὀστέων κατά τινα
ἰδίαν κρᾶσιν. * * ὧδε καὶ φλέβας· * παρα-
[σκευάζ]ει δύο, τὴν μὲν εἰς δεξιὰ τὴν
15 δὲ εἰς εὐώνυμα, ὧν τῆς μὲν δεξιᾶς
τὰς ἀποσχίδας καταπλέκειν τὰ εὐώνυμα μέρη, * τῆς δὲ εὐωνύμου τὰ δεξιά.
κοιλίας τε δύο ὑπάρχειν, ὧν τὴν μὲν ἄνω,
τὴν δὲ κάτω· καὶ τὴν κάτω ὑποκεῖσθαι
20 πρὸς ὑποδοχὴν τῶν περιττωμάτων.
περὶ ταύτηι δὲ γενέσθαι μακρόν τε
καὶ εἱλιγμένον ἔντερον, ἵνα μὴ ἡ λαμβανομένη
τροφὴ ῥαιδίως καταφέρηται, ἀλλὰ ὑπομένηι
ποσοὺς χρόνους. * ὡς γὰρ τῶν κατ᾽ εὐθυωρί-
25 αν κειμένων ποταμῶν τὰ ῥεύματά ἐστιν
οὐκ ἀνάσχετα, τῶν δὲ σκολιῶν ἠπιώ-
τερα διὰ τὸ ἐνκόπτεσθαι, οὕτως εἰ μὲν βρα-
χὺ ἐγένετο τὸ ἔντερον τὸ πρὸς τὴν κάτω
κοιλίαν καὶ εὐθύ, κἂν ἐφέρετο ῥαδίως
30 ἡ τροφή. * ἐπεὶ δὲ σκολιόν τέ ἐστιν καὶ πο-
λύμηκες, ταύτηι ἐπιμένει πολλοὺς χρόνους.
καὶ περὶ μὲν τοῦ σώματος τοσαῦτα.
λέγει δὲ καὶ περὶ τῆς ψυχῆς, ὡς τρι-
μερής ἐστιν, καὶ τὸ μέν τι αὐτῆς ἐστιν λογικόν,
35 τὸ δὲ θυμικόν, τὸ δὲ ἐπιθυμητι-
κόν. καὶ τὸ μὲν λογικὸν ἀπολείπει περὶ

4. Plato, *Tim.* 74a–b.
11. Plato, *Tim.* 74d.
13. Plato, *Tim.* 77c–e.
20. Plato, *Tim.* 72e–73a.
36. Plato, *Tim.* 45a–b.

8. After ἔξωθεν D. thinks κλᾶν or κάμπτειν has been lost.

XVI stomach does not bring forth a refined intelligence". ∗ ∗ The bones, says

Plato, are solid, so that they can serve as a support; while joints have

been made for them, that the limbs may be drawn up and bent. ∗ For

them sinews outside ∗ ∗ [mitigate] the hardness of the bones for the sake

of voluntary movements ∗ ∗ and flesh as a shield against cold and

heat. ∗ The sinews are composed of unleavened flesh and of bones

compounded according to a special formula. ∗ ∗ thus too the veins. ∗

He arranges two, one to the right, the other to the left, the left parts

of which entwine the branches of the right vein ∗ and the right parts

the branches of the left. There are, he says, two bellies, upper and lower.

The lower lies beneath to serve as a reservoir for the residues. Around

it has been placed a long and winding intestine, in order that the nutri-

ment taken may not easily sink but remain for specified periods of time. ∗

For as the streams of rivers that flow straight are irresistible, but those

of winding streams are more gentle because impeded, so if the intestine

leading to the lower belly had been made short and straight, the nutriment

also would move easily. ∗ But since it is winding and very long, the nutri-

ment for that reason remains there for long periods of time. So much

for the body. Plato also treats of the soul, saying that it is tripartite, with

a rational part, a spirited part and an appetitive part. The rational part

12. ἀζύμου. See XV. 35 and *Tim.* 74d.

XVI   τοὺς κατὰ τὴν κεφαλὴν τόπους· εὐφυὴς γὰρ
αὕτη γίνεται πρὸς παραδοχὴν τοῦ ἡγεμονικοῦ·
τὸ δὲ θυμικὸν ἔταξεν περὶ τὴν καρδίαν,
40   οὐ πόρρω μὲν τεταγμένον τοῦ λογικοῦ,
ὑποτεταγμένον δὲ τῶι λογικῶι,
ἵνα δὴ καὶ ὑπήκοον αὐτῶι γίνηται. * τὸ μέντοι
γ̄ τὸ ἐπιθυμητικὸν ἔταξεν μεταξὺ διαφράγματος καὶ ὀμφαλοῦ. * ἐπέστησεν
45   δὲ τὸ ἧπαρ τῆι ἐπιθυμίαι κάτοχον, ἵνα

XVII   τὰς ἐπιθυμίας ταπεινοῖ τοῖς εἰδώλοις,
τόν τε πνεύμονα πρὸς τῆι καρδίαι, ἧς ὀξεῖα
ἡ φύσις, μαλακὸν τάσσει σπόγγον, ἵνα
ἡ καρδία, φησίν, πυκινοκείνητος οὖσα ἁλ-
5   λομένη μὴ ῥηγνύηται. * τὸν δὲ σπλῆνα
λέγει ἐγμαγεῖον εἶναι ἕτοιμον ἀεὶ παρακείμενον,
ἐπειδήπερ νοσοῦντι μὲν τῶι ἥπατι καὶ
αὐτὸς συννοσεῖ καὶ συναύξεται, τῶι δὲ
ὑγιαίνοντι συνυγιαίνει, ἀεὶ ἄγων αὐτὸ
10   εἰς τὸ κατὰ φύσιν. καὶ περὶ τῆς ψυχῆς
δὲ ταῦτα. * λέγει δὲ γίνεσθαι τὰς νόσους
τριχῶς, ἢ παρὰ τὰ στοιχεῖα ἢ παρὰ τὴν
γένεσιν τῶν σωμάτων ἢ παρὰ τὰ τούτων
περισσώματα. καὶ παρὰ μὲν τὰ στοιχεῖα
15   γίνονται νόσοι, ὅταν ἢ πλείονα γένη τὸ
εἶδος μεταβάληι ἢ ἐν ἀνοικείωι καθί-
σηι· καὶ γὰρ πλείονα γενόμενα ταῦτα
τὰ στοιχεῖα νόσους κατασκευάζει διὰ
τὸ πλῆθος· * καὶ μὴν καὶ ἐγβάντα τοῦ
20   οἰκείου εἴδους πάλι ἐνποιεῖται ἑτέροις.

XVI. 39. Plato, *Tim.* 69 d–70 a.
42. Plato, *Tim.* 70 d–71 b.
XVII. 2. Plato, *Tim.* 70 c–d.
4. Hippocrates, *de articulis* (IV. 124, 15 L.): ἠνάγκασται γὰρ (ἡ κληίς)
πυκινοκίνητος εἶναι (cf. Galen, XVIII. A 415 K.).
5. Plato, *Tim.* 72 c–d.
11. Plato, *Tim.* 81 e–82 e.

XVI. 45. κατεχον or κατοχον P.: κάτοπτρον should be restored from
Timaeus, 71 b.
XVII. 15. I suggest adding ἢ ἢ after γένη: Cornford γένη⟨ται καί (or ἤ)⟩.

XVI he assigns to the regions about the head, for the head proves adapted by nature for the reception of the governing part. The spirited part he stationed around the heart; it is stationed not far from the intellectual part but underneath it, in order of course that it may be subject to it. * The third, the appetitive part, however, he stationed between the midriff and the navel. * He set the liver to hold down appetite, XVII so that it might abate appetites by its images, while by the heart, whose nature is quick, he places the soft sponge of the lungs, so that the heart (so he says) with its rapid motion may not be ruptured when it jumps. * The spleen he says is a towel always lying ready beside it, since when the liver is diseased the spleen too is diseased and enlarges with it, and when it is well the spleen is well with it, always leading it towards the natural condition. So much for the soul. * Diseases, he says, come about in three ways: (1) because of the elements, (2) because of the formation of bodies and (3) because of their residues. Diseases occur because of the elements when there are too many kinds or when they change their form or settle in an unsuitable place, for these elements when they become too many cause diseases through their number, * and further they depart from the suitable form and are made again in

XVI. 45. If for κάτοχον we read κάτοπτρον: "he set the liver over appetite to be its mirror". The student again misheard the lecturer.

XVII. 4. "So he says": not in *Timaeus*, nor is πυκινοκίνητος.

11–17. In the *Timaeus* (82 a) we are told that diseases arise (1) from an unnatural prevalence or deficiency of the elements, or (2) from their migration from their own proper place to an alien one; or (3) since there are several varieties of fire, etc., from any bodily part's taking in an unsuitable variety.

The text of P. gives not three possibilities but two only. Of these the former, "when several kinds change their forms", is not in Plato as it stands, for the change of one element only to an unsuitable variety is sufficient to cause disease. If we assume that ἢ ἤ has fallen out after γένη, the text of P. becomes a fair paraphrase of the passage in the *Timaeus*. Cornford's γένη⟨ται καὶ⟩ is perhaps better, because of καὶ γὰρ πλείονα γενόμενα ταῦτα (l. 17).

13. τούτων: the elements.

15. I assume in the translation that my emendation is correct.

19. πλῆθος, possibly "bulk".

XVII

ἀλλὰ γὰρ ὡς ὁμοίως καὶ ἐν ἀνοικείοις τόποις ταχθέντα νόσους ἐπιφέρει πολλὰς
τοῦτο τὸ δὴ ἐν ἀνοικείωι τόπωι γινόμενον εἶδος.
καὶ παρὰ μὲν τὴν τῶν στοιχείων διάθεσιν
25 οὕτως συνίστανται αἱ νόσοι. * * παρὰ δὲ αὖ
τὴν γένεσιν τῶν σωμάτων γίνονται νόσοι τινὲς τοιούτων,
οἷον ἡ σὰρξ λαμβάνει τὴν γένεσιν
ἐξ αἵματος πεπηγότος καὶ συνεστα-
μένου, τὰ δὲ νεῦρα ἀποτελεῖται ἐκ τῶν
30 †ε†ἰνῶν τοῦ αἵματος. ταύτηι δὲ ἀναιρε-
θεισῶν τῶν τοῦ αἵματος ἰνῶν ἄπηκτον
διαμένει λοιπὸν τὸ αἷμα, ὃ γίνεται ἐν ἐκείνηι,
ὅτι ἡ μὲν σὰρξ ἐξ αἵματος λαμβάνει
τὴν γένεσιν, τὰ δὲ νεῦρα ἐκ τῶν τοῦ
35 αἵματος ἰνῶν. "ταύτηι δὴ συνέχεται,
φησίν, καὶ τρέφεται τὰ σώματα ταῦτα
πρὸς τῆς πειμελῆς, τηκομένης
αὐτῆς καὶ διὰ τῶν ἀραιοτήτων τῶν ὀστέων
ἐπιχορηγουμένης καὶ τρεφούσης
40 τὰ ὀστέα. ὅταν μὲν οὖν οὕτως γίνηται ἡ τῶν σωμάτων γένεσις, κατὰ φύσιν ἔχει τὸ ζῶιον·
ὅταν δὲ μὴ οὕτως γίνηται, ἀλλ᾽ ἐνηλλαγμένως
ἡ γένεσις, νόσους ἐπιφέρει." καὶ περὶ τὴν
γένεσιν δὲ τῶν σωμάτων οὕτως. * * παρὰ δὲ
45 τὰ περιττώματα συνίστανται τριχῶς
αἱ νόσοι, ἢ παρὰ τὰς φύσας τὰς ἐκ τῶν πε-

XVIII

ριττωμάτων ἢ παρὰ χολὴν ἢ φλέγμα· διὰ
γὰρ ταῦτα τὰ τρία καὶ κοινῆι καὶ ἰδίαι γίνονται
νόσοι. καὶ γὰρ ἓν μόνον αὐτῶν νόσους ἐπιφέρει
καὶ δύο συνάμφω συνελθόντα πάλι νό-
5 σους κατασκευάζει. * ὡς ὁμοίως δὲ καὶ διὰ
τὰ τρία συγκατοισθέντα αἱ νόσοι ἀπο-
τελοῦνται. καὶ ἡ μὲν τοῦ Πλάτωνος
δόξα περὶ νόσων ἐν τούτοις. * * Φιλόλαος

XVII. 44. Plato, *Tim.* 84c–e.

XVII. 22. Only the -ς of πολλὰς remains. Perhaps τινὰς (D).
23. Hackforth would insert καὶ before τοῦτο.
46. For ἐκ τῶν Edelstein would read μετά.

XVII different forms. In fact just as elements stationed in unsuitable places bring on many diseases, so does this form, of course, when it arises in an unsuitable place. This is the way those diseases come about that are due to the condition of the elements. * * Then again the formation of the following kinds of body gives rise to certain diseases; for example flesh receives its formation from fixed and solidified blood, and the sinews are fashioned out of the fibrine of the blood. And thus if the fibrine of the blood be destroyed, the blood that is found in flesh (?) remains behind without solidifying, because flesh receives its formation from blood and the sinews from the fibrine of the blood. "Thus then these bodies," he says, "are bound together and are nourished by the fat, which itself melting and being supplied through the porousness of the bones, nourishes the bones. So when the formation of the bodies proceeds on these lines, the creature is in a natural condition; but when the formation is not so, but contrariwise, diseases are brought on."

So much for the formation of bodies. * * Residues produce diseases XVIII in three ways—(1) because of the gases arising from the residues, (2) because of bile or (3) because of phlegm. For it is because of these three that diseases arise both in general and in particular instances. In fact one alone of them brings on diseases and the union of two together also causes diseases. * Similarly a conjunction of the three likewise produces diseases. Such is the view of Plato about diseases. * *

XVII. 32. The context seems to require ἐκείνη to refer to σάρξ, although the noun is six lines back and occurs again immediately afterwards. Linguistic carelessness again.

35–43. Though given as a quotation this passage is a free paraphrase of *Tim.* 82 d, e.

40–43. From *Timaeus*, 82 c we learn that the worst diseases result when growth as it were goes backward (ὅταν ἀνάπαλιν ἡ γένεσις τούτων πορεύηται, cf. ὅταν ἐναντίως in 82 e). This makes it quite clear what Anonymus meant by ἐνηλλαγμένως, although it is hard to see why Plato's ἀνάπαλιν or ἐναντίως should have been discarded for a much clumsier word. See F. M. Cornford, *Plato's Cosmology*, p. 336.

XVIII
10

δὲ ὁ Κροτωνιάτης συνεστάναι φησὶν τὰ ἡμέτερα σώματα ἐκ θερμοῦ. ἀμέτοχα γὰρ αὐτὰ εἶναι
ψυχροῦ, [ὑπομι]μνήσκων ἀπό τινων τοιούτων·
τὸ σπέρμ[α εἶναι θερ]μόν, κατασκευαστικὸν δὲ
τοῦτο τοῦ ζώιου· καὶ ὁ τόπος δέ, εἰς ὃν
ἡ καταβολή — μήτρα δὲ αὕτη — ἐστὶν θερμοτέρα

15

καὶ ἐοικυῖα ἐκείνωι· τὸ δὲ ἐοικός τινι τἀτὸ δύναται, ὧι ἔοικεν·
ἐπεὶ δὲ τὸ κατα-
σκευάζον ἀμέτοχόν ἐστιν ψυχροῦ καὶ ὁ τόπος
δέ, ἐν ὧι ἡ καταβολή, ἀμέτοχός ἐστιν ψυχροῦ,
δῆλον ὅτι καὶ τὸ κατασκευαζόμενον ζῶιον
τοιοῦτον γίνεται. * εἰς δὲ τούτου τὴν

20

κατασκευὴν ὑπομνήσει προσχρῆται τοιαύ-
τηι· μετὰ γὰρ τὴν ἔκτεξιν εὐθέως †το†
τὸ ζῶιον ἐπισπᾶται τὸ ἐκτὸς πνεῦμα
ψυχρὸν ὄν· εἶτα πάλιν καθαπερεὶ χρέος
ἐκπέμπει αὐτό. * διὰ τοῦτο δὴ καὶ ὄρεξις

25

τοῦ ἐκτὸς πνεύματος, ἵνα τῆι
ἐπεισάκτωι τοῦ πνεύματος ὁλκῆι θερμότερα ὑπάρχοντα τὰ ἡμέτερα σώματα πρὸς αὐτοῦ
καταψύχηται. * καὶ τὴν μὲν σύστασιν
τῶν ἡμετέρων σωμάτων ἐν τούτοις φησίν. * *

30

λέγει δὲ γίνεσθαι τὰς νόσους διά τε χολὴν
καὶ αἷμα καὶ φλέγμα, ἀρχὴν δὲ γίνεσθαι
τῶν νόσων ταῦτα· ἀποτελεῖσθαι
δέ φησιν τὸ μὲν αἷμα παχὺ μὲν ἔσω παρα-
θλιβομένης τῆς σαρκός, * λεπτὸν

35

δὲ γίνεσθαι διαιρουμένων τῶν ἐν τῆι σαρκὶ ἀγγείων·
τὸ δὲ φλέγμα συνίστασθαι ἀπὸ τῶν ὄμ-
βρων φησίν. λέγει δὲ τὴν χολὴν ἰχῶρα
εἶναι τῆς σαρκός. * παράδοξόν τε αὐτὸς
ἀνὴρ ἐπὶ τούτου κεινεῖ· λέγει γὰρ μηδὲ τε-

40

τάχθαι ἐπὶ τῶι ἥπατι χολήν, ἰχῶρα μέντοι τῆς σαρκὸς εἶναι τὴν χολήν. * τό τ᾽ αὖ
φλέγμα τῶν πλείστων ψυχρὸν †θερμον† εἶναι λεγόν-
των αὐτὸς θερμὸν τῆι φύσει ὑποτί-

---

10. P. has αμετα or αμεγα. K. would read ἀμιγῆ, D. ἀμέτοχα (citing XVI. 17).
19. ἔσται K.

XVIII. 20 Philolaus of Croton says that our bodies are composed of heat.

They have, he says, no part in cold, and mentions as evidence for this view facts like the following. The seed, constructive of the living creature, is warm, and the place in which it is deposited, that is to say the womb, is like the seed, being warmer still. What is like a thing has the same quality as the thing it resembles. Since the constructive agent has no part in cold, and the place in which it is deposited has no part in cold, it is plain that the living creature that is constructed has also no part in cold. * About the construction of it he mentions further the following particulars. Immediately after birth the creature inhales the external air, which is cold. Then it discharges it again like a debt. * Appetite too for the external air has as its object that our bodies, being too hot, through the drawing in of breath from without may be cooled thereby. * The composition of our bodies he describes in these terms. * * Diseases arise, he holds, through bile, blood and phlegm, and these are the origin of diseases. The blood, he says, is rendered thick when the flesh is compressed inwards; * it becomes thin when the vessels in the flesh are broken up. Phlegm, he says, is made from the rains. He also says that bile is a serum of flesh. * The same man is in this matter guilty of an absurdity. For he makes bile a serum of flesh, but denies that it has its station in the liver. * Again, while most say that phlegm is cold, he lays it down that it is by nature hot,

10. See [Hippocrates], *Fleshes*, ch. II: L. VIII. 584.
36, 37. Perhaps "from the rainy season". Or is ὄμβροι merely "water"?
39. For μηδέ see p. 33.
40, 41. The παράδοξον is apparently denying the obvious connection between bile and the liver.

XVIII

θεται· ἀπὸ γὰρ τοῦ φλέγειν φλέγμα εἰρῆσθαι·
45 ταύτηι δὲ καὶ τὰ φλεγμαίνοντα
μετοχῆι τοῦ φλέγματος φλεγμαί-
νει. καὶ ταῦτα μὲν δὴ ἀρχὰς τῶν νόσων
ὑποτίθεται, * συνεργὰ δὲ ὑπερβολάς
τε θερμασίας, τροφῆς, καταψύξεως καὶ

XIX

ἐνδείας τούτων ἢ τῶν τούτοις παραπλησίων. * * ὁ δὲ
Πόλυβος ἐξ ἑνὸς μὲν στοιχείου οὐ λέγει

XVIII. 44. Galen, II. 130 K.: Πρόδικος δ' ἐν τῷ Περὶ φύσεως ἀνθρώπου
γράμματι τὸ συγκεκαυμένον καὶ οἷον ὑπερωπτημένον ἐν τοῖς χυμοῖς ὀνο-
μάζων φλέγμα παρὰ τὸ πεφλέχθαι, τῇ λέξει μὲν ἑτέρως χρῆται,
φυλάττει μέντοι τὸ πρᾶγμα κατὰ ταὐτὸ τοῖς ἄλλοις. τὴν δ' ἐν τοῖς
ὀνόμασι τἀνδρὸς τούτου καινοτομίαν ἱκανῶς ἐνδείκνυται καὶ Πλάτων.
ἀλλὰ τοῦτό γε τὸ πρὸς ἁπάντων ἀνθρώπων ὀνομαζόμενον φλέγμα τὸ
λευκὸν τὴν χρόαν, ὃ βλένναν ὀνομάζει Πρόδικος, ὁ ψυχρὸς καὶ ὑγρὸς
χυμός ἐστιν οὗτος καὶ πλεῖστος τοῖς τε γέρουσι καὶ τοῖς ὁπωσδήποτε
ψυγεῖσιν ἀθροίζεται καὶ οὐδεὶς οὐδὲ μαινόμενος ἂν ἄλλο τι ἢ ψυχρὸν καὶ
ὑγρὸν εἴποι ἂν αὐτόν.

XIX. 2.   Hippocrates, περὶ φύσιος ἀνθρώπου, 3 (VI. 38, 5 L.): πῶς εἰκὸς
ἀπὸ ἑνός τι γεννηθῆναι ὅτε οὐδ' ἀπὸ τῶν πλειόνων γίνεται, ἢν μὴ τύχῃ
καλῶς ἔχοντα τῆς κρήσιος τῆς πρὸς ἄλληλα; ἀνάγκη τοίνυν τῆς φύσιος
τοιαύτης ὑπαρχούσης καὶ τῶν ἄλλων πάντων καὶ τῆς τοῦ ἀνθρώπου μὴ ἐν
εἶναι τὸν ἄνθρωπον, ἀλλ' ἕκαστον τῶν ξυμβαλλομένων ἐς τὴν γένεσιν ἔχειν
τὴν δύναμιν ἐν τῷ σώματι οἵηνπερ συνεβάλετο. καὶ πάλιν γε ἀνάγκη
ἀναχωρεῖν ἐς τὴν ἑωυτοῦ φύσιν ἕκαστον τελευτῶντος τοῦ σώματος τοῦ
ἀνθρώπου τό τε ὑγρὸν πρὸς τὸ ὑγρὸν καὶ τὸ ξηρὸν πρὸς τὸ ξηρὸν καὶ τὸ
θερμὸν πρὸς τὸ θερμὸν καὶ τὸ ψυχρὸν πρὸς τὸ ψυχρόν. τοιαύτη δὲ καὶ
τῶν ζώων ἐστὶν ἡ φύσις καὶ τῶν ἄλλων πάντων· γίνεταί τε ὁμοίως πάντα
καὶ τελευτᾷ ὁμοίως πάντα. συνίσταταί τε γὰρ αὐτῶν ἡ φύσις ἀπὸ τούτων
τῶν εἰρημένων πάντων καὶ τελευτᾷ κατὰ τὰ εἰρημένα ἐς τὸ αὐτὸ ὅθεν περ
συνέστη ἕκαστον, ἐνταῦθα οὖν καὶ ἀπεχώρησεν. Ibidem, 2 (VI. 34, 8 L.):
τῶν δὲ ἰητρῶν οἱ μέν τινες λέγουσιν, ὡς ἄνθρωπος αἷμά ἐστιν, οἱ δὲ αὐτῶν
χολήν φασιν εἶναι τὸν ἄνθρωπον, ἔνιοι δέ τινες φλέγμα· ἐπίλογον δὲ ποιέονται
καὶ οὗτοι πάντες τὸν αὐτόν· ἐν γὰρ εἶναί φασιν, ὅ τι ἕκαστος αὐτῶν βούλεται
ὀνομάσας καὶ τοῦτο μεταλλάσσειν τὴν ἰδέην καὶ τὴν δύναμιν ἀναγκαζόμενον
ὑπό τε τοῦ θερμοῦ καὶ τοῦ ψυχροῦ καὶ γίνεσθαι γλυκὺ καὶ πικρὸν καὶ λευκὸν
καὶ μέλαν καὶ παντοῖον. ἐμοὶ δὲ οὐδέν τι δοκεῖ ταῦτα οὕτως ἔχειν· οἱ μὲν
οὖν πλεῖστοι τοιαῦτά τινα καὶ ἐγγύτατα τούτων ἀποφαίνονται. ἐγὼ δέ
φημι· εἰ ἓν ἦν ὥνθρωπος οὐδέποτ' ἂν ἄλγεεν· οὐδὲ γὰρ ἦν ὑφ' οὗ ἀλγήσειεν
ἐν ἐών· εἰ δ' οὖν καὶ ἀλγήσειεν, ἀνάγκη καὶ τὸ ἰώμενον ἓν εἶναι· νῦν δὲ
πολλά· πολλὰ γάρ ἐστιν ἐν τῷ σώματι ἐνεόντα, ἃ ὅταν ὑπ' ἀλλήλων παρὰ
φύσιν θερμαίνηταί τε καὶ ψύχηται καὶ ξηραίνηταί τε καὶ ὑγραίνηται νόσους
τίκτει.

XIX. 1.   τούτων ἢ added by M. Fränkel.

XVIII "phlegm" being derived from *phlegein* (to burn). Wherefore too it is by participation in phlegm that inflamed parts are inflamed (*phlegmainein*). These are the things that Philolaus postulates as the causes of diseases. * Contributory, he says, are excesses of heat, of nutriment, XIX. 21 of chill, and also defects of these or of things like these. * *

Polybus says that our bodies are not composed of one element, but

XIX. 2–18. This part of *Nature of Man* is here attributed to Polybus, but in VII. 15 ff. ch. 9 of that work is assigned to Hippocrates. The work is composite (see Fredrich's dissertation), and different parts may in ancient times have been attributed to different authors.

XIX τὰ ἡμέτερα σώματα συνεστάναι, τὴν δὲ
αὐτὴν φύσιν ὁμοίως πᾶσιν εἶναι, ἥπερ ἐκ
5 ψυχροῦ τε καὶ θερμοῦ, οὐ χωρὶς ὄντων τούτων,
ἀλλὰ κεκραμένων αὐτῶν, συνέστηκεν· μετα-
βαλὸν δὲ θάτερον θατέρωι νόσον ἀπο-
τελεῖν. * δευτέραν δὲ ἀποτελεῖσθαι
τῶν σωμάτων μεταβολὴν ἀπὸ αἵματός τε
10 καὶ φλέγματος καὶ χολῆς ξανθῆς τε
καὶ μελαίνης. ἀπὸ δυνάμεως γὰρ πάντων
τούτων ἢ ἑνὸς αὐτῶν γίνεσθαι ταύτην τὴν
μεταβολήν, ἢ κατὰ τὸν αὐτὸν τόπον γινομένης τῆς
συμμίξεως κατὰ φύσιν γίνεται· ἐὰν δ' ἐν τῶι
15 σώματι †γινεται† χωρισθῆι τι ἀπὸ τῶν ἄλλων,
νόσους γίνεσθαι. νοσεῖν δὲ καὶ ἀφ' ὧνπερ ἐχω-
ρίσθη†σαν† τόπων καὶ εἰς οὕσπερ ἐχώ-
ρησεν. Μενεκράτης δὲ ὁ Ζεὺς ἐπι-
κληθεὶς ἐν Ἰατρικῆι δεῖξίν τινα τῶν
20 σωμάτων ἐκτιθέμενος καὶ μέλλων αἰτιολογεῖν
τὰ πάθη, πρότερον περὶ τῶν ποιοτήτων
πολυπραγμονῶν τῶν σωμάτων, συνεστάναι
λέγει τὰ σώματα ἐκ τῶν τεσσάρων
στοιχείων, β μὲν θερμῶν, β δὲ ψυχρῶν· καὶ
25 θερμῶν μὲν αἵματος καὶ χολῆς, ψυχρῶν
δὲ πνεύματος καὶ φλέγματος. * καὶ
τούτων μὲν δὴ μὴ στασιαζόντων, ἀλλ' εὐκρό-

---

8. Hippocrates, περὶ φύσιος ἀνθρώπου, 4 (VI. 38, 19 L.; cf. Galen,
de plac. Hipp. et Plat. p. 677, 13 ff. M.): τὸ δὲ σῶμα τοῦ ἀνθρώπου ἔχει
ἐν ἑωυτῷ αἷμα καὶ φλέγμα καὶ χολὴν ξανθήν τε καὶ μέλαιναν, καὶ ταῦτά
ἐστιν αὐτῷ ἡ φύσις τοῦ σώματος καὶ δι' αὐτὰ ἀλγεῖ καὶ ὑγιαίνει. ὑγιαίνει
μὲν οὖν μάλιστα, ὅταν μετρίως ἔχῃ ταῦτα τῆς πρὸς ἄλληλα δυνάμιος καὶ
τοῦ πλήθεος καὶ μάλιστα μεμιγμένα ᾖ. ἀλγεῖ δ' ὅταν τούτων τι ἔλασσον
ἢ πλέον χωρισθῇ ἐν τῷ σώματι καὶ μὴ κεκρημένον ᾖ τοῖσι πᾶσιν. ἀνάγκη
γάρ, ὅταν τούτων τι χωρισθῇ καὶ ἐφ' ἑωυτοῦ στῇ, οὐ μόνον τοῦτο τὸ χωρίον,
ἔνθεν ἐξέστη, ἐπίνοσον γίγνεσθαι, ἀλλὰ καὶ ἔνθα ἂν στῇ καὶ ἐπιχυθῇ ὑπερ-
πιμπλάμενον ὀδύνην τε καὶ πόνον παρέχειν. καὶ γὰρ ὅταν τι τούτων ἔξω
τοῦ σώματος ἐκρυῇ πλέον τοῦ ἐπιπολάζοντος, ὀδύνην παρέχει ἡ κένωσις·
ἤν τ' αὖ πάλιν εἴσω ποιήσηται τὴν κένωσιν καὶ τὴν μετάστασιν καὶ τὴν
ἀπόκρισιν ἀπὸ τῶν ἄλλων, πολλὴ αὐτῷ ἀνάγκη διπλὴν τὴν ὀδύνην παρέχειν
κατὰ τὰ εἰρημένα, ἔνθεν τε ἐξέστη καὶ ἔνθα ὑπερέβαλεν.

---

7. Read θατέρου for θατέρωι.

XIX that they all alike have the same nature, which is composed out of the cold and the hot, not separated, but blended. A change of one for the other produces disease. * A second change in bodies is brought about proceeding from blood, phlegm, yellow bile and black bile. For from the power of all these or of one of them this change occurs, which, if the mixture occurs in the same place, occurs naturally; but if in the body one be separated from the others, diseases occur. Both the places from which and those to which the separation occurs are diseased.

22 Menecrates surnamed Zeus when setting forth in his book *Medicine* an explanation of bodies, and when about to trace the causes of affections, first goes at some length into the qualities of bodies, saying that bodies are composed out of the four elements, two of which are hot, and two cold, the hot being blood and bile, the cold, breath and phlegm. * And when these do not disagree, but are in a state of harmony, the

6. "Blended": perhaps, "compounded".

9. μεταβολὴν is a difficult word here. It is apparently used in two senses: (*a*) the change occurring when the four elements combine; (*b*) the change occurring when one element separates out from the others in combination.

14. A most difficult sentence. It apparently means: (*a*) when the powers of the four elements combine in one place, the result is a "change" κατὰ φύσιν; (*b*) but the "change" may come from the power of one element. Then, as the next two sentences say, there is removal of this element from one place to another, both of which places thus become diseased.

It would have been clearer if μεταβολή had not been used in sense (*a*), which would be more clearly expressed by κρᾶσις or even σύστασις.

Cornford thinks that in this passage μεταβολή means "derangement".

XIX

τως διακειμένων ὑγιαίνειν τὸ σῶμα,
δυσκρότως δὲ ἐχόντων νοσεῖν. τότε

30 γὰρ ἐκθεῖν ἐκ τῶν ἡμετέρων σωμάτων φλέγ-
ματα, δοθίονας καὶ τὰ τούτοις ὅμοια.
καὶ κατάρρους δὲ ἐκ τῆς ὑπερβολῆς τοῦ
φλέγματος διαφόρους γίνεσθαι......
οὔμενον γάρ, φησίν, ἐν τῶι σώματι.......εἰ-

35 σιόντι δὲ φλέγματι τὸ κειθα......
νομενεισ. αιπο . . την κ...........
ἐμμεῖναν δὲ τοῦτο πυρρὰν χολὴν
ἀπογεννᾶι. ἐμμείνασα δὲ αὕτη
καὶ παλαιωθεῖσα μέλαιναν ἀπογεννᾶι

40 χολήν. * ἢν δὲ καὶ παλαιωθεῖσαν
καὶ ὑπέρχολον γενομένην δέχηταί τι,
ὅπου ἂν τύχηι, μέρος καὶ κυῆι, οὐδέν φησιν
ἀγαθὸν ἐργάζεσθαι· οἰσθεῖσα μὲν γὰρ
ἐπὶ ἰσχία ἰσχιαδικὴν ἐμποιεῖ,

45 ἐπὶ δὲ τὸν πνεύμονα περιπνευμονίαν,
ἐπὶ δὲ τὰς πλευρὰς πλευρεῖτιν,
ἐπὶ δὲ τὰ σπλάγχνα οἰσθεῖσα
καῦσον ἀπεργάζεται· τοιαῦτα δὲ πολλὰ

XX

καὶ διάφορα γίνεται πάθη. * * ὁ δὲ Αἰγινήτης
Πέτρων συνεστάναι φησὶν τὰ ἡμέτερα
σώματα ἐκ δισσῶν στοιχείων, ψυχροῦ
τε καὶ θερμοῦ, ἐφ' ἑτέρωι δὲ τούτων

5 ἀπολείπει τι ἀντίστοιχον, τῶι μὲν
θερμῶι τὸ ξηρόν, τῶι δὲ ψυχρῶι τὸ ὑγρόν.
καὶ ἐγ μὲν δὴ τούτων συνεστάναι τὰ σώματα.
φησὶν δὲ γίνεσθαι τὰς νόσους ἁπλῶς
μὲν διὰ τὰς περιττώσεις τῆς τροφῆς·

10 ὅταν, ἃ σύμμετρα, ἡ κοιλία μὴ λα-
βοῦσα, πλείω δέ, μὴ κατεργάσηται
αὐτά, συμβαίνει νόσους γίνεσθαι. ἢ ἀπὸ τῶν
στοιχείων τῶν προειρημένων, ὅταν ἀνώ-
μαλα ἦι, νόσους ἀπεργάζεται. περὶ

15 δὲ τῆς διαφορᾶς τῆς κατὰ τὰς νόσους οὐδὲν διακριβοῖ. περὶ δὲ τῆς
χολῆς ἰδιώτερον παθολογεῖ. φησὶν γὰρ αὐ-

XIX. 33, 34. Probably ἀλλοιούμενον.

XIX body is healthy; when they are not in harmony, it is diseased. For then there are expelled from our bodies phlegms, boils and the like. Catarrhs also of various kinds arise from the excess of phlegm. For changing, he says, in the body.....having remained there this produces red bile. This having remained and grown stale produces black bile. * And if when it has become stale and very bitter there receive it, wherever it may chance, some part of the body which becomes pregnant, then, he says, no good results. For if it be carried to the hips it brings on lumbago; to the lungs, pneumonia; to the ribs, pleurisy; and if it be carried to the bowels it results in ardent fever. Many different affections occur of this kind. * *

XX. 23 Petron of Aegina says that our bodies are composed of a pair of elements, the cold and the hot, and to each of these he assigns a partner, to the hot the dry and to the cold the moist, and out of these are our bodies composed. And he says that diseases may arise simply through the residues of nutriment. Whenever the belly taking in nutriment not commensurate with it, but overmuch, cannot digest it, the result is that diseases occur. He also derives diseases from the aforesaid elements, when they are disproportionate. But about the different kinds of diseases he gives no details. As to bile, however, he holds pathological

XIX. 48. καῦσος, either remittent malaria or typhoid. See the Loeb *Hippocrates*, I. lvi.
XX. 1. For Petron see p. 16.
5. ἀντίστοιχον, perhaps "correlative".
14. The subject of ἀπεργάζεται is Petron.

XX   τὴν ὑπὸ τῶν νόσων †σωματων† κατασκευάζεσθαι.

οἱ μὲν γὰρ ἄλλοι ἀπὸ τῆς χολῆς λέγουσι

20   γίνεσθαι τὰς νόσους, οὗτος δὲ ἀπὸ τῶν

νόσων τὴν χολήν. καὶ σχεδὸν οὗτος ὡς

ὁ Φιλόλαος οἴεται μὴ εἶναι ἐν ἡμῖν χολὴν ἢ

ἀχρείαν. καὶ κατὰ μὲν ταῦτα συνηγόρευ-

σεν τῶι Φιλολάωι, κατὰ δὲ τἆλλα †αυτονει†.

25   Φιλιστίων δ᾽ οἴεται ἐκ δ ἰδεῶν συνεστά-

ναι ἡμᾶς, τοῦτ᾽ ἔστιν ἐκ δ στοιχείων· πυρός,

ἀέρος, ὕδατος, γῆς. εἶναι δὲ καὶ ἑκάστου δυνάμεις,

τοῦ μὲν πυρὸς τὸ θερμόν, τοῦ δὲ ἀέρος

τὸ ψυχρόν, τοῦ δὲ ὕδατος τὸ ὑγρόν,

30   τῆς δὲ γῆς τὸ ξηρόν. * * τὰς δὲ νόσους γίνεσθαι

πολυτρόπως κατ᾽ αὐτόν, ὡς δὲ τύπωι

καὶ γενικώτερον εἰπεῖν τριχῶς· ἢ γὰρ παρὰ

τὰ στοιχεῖα ἢ παρὰ τὴν τῶν σωμάτων διά-

θεσιν ἢ παρὰ τὰ ἐκτός. * παρὰ μὲν οὖν τὰ

35   στοιχεῖα, ἐπειδὰν πλεονάσηι τὸ θερμὸν

καὶ τὸ ὑγρόν, ἢ ἐπειδὰν μεῖον γένηται

καὶ ἀ†υ†μαυρὸν τὸ θερμόν. * * παρὰ δὲ τὰ

ἐκτὸς γ̄· ἢ γὰρ ὑπὸ τραυμάτων καὶ ἑλκῶν

ἢ ὑπὸ ὑπερβολῆς θάλπους, ψύχους, τῶν ὁμοίων,

40   ἢ ὑπὸ μεταβολῆς θερμοῦ εἰς ψυχρὸν

ἢ ψυχροῦ εἰς θερμὸν ἢ τροφῆς εἰς τὸ

ἀνοίκειον καὶ διεφθορός. * παρὰ δὲ τὴν

τῶν σωμάτων διάθεσιν οὕτως· "ὅταν γάρ, φησίν, εὐ-

πνοῆι ὅλον τὸ σῶμα καὶ διεξίηι ἀκω-

45   λύτως τὸ πνεῦμα, ὑγίεια γίνεται· οὐ γὰρ μόνον κατὰ

τὸ στόμα καὶ τοὺς μυκτῆρας ἡ ἀνα-

πνοὴ γίνεται, ἀλλὰ καὶ καθ᾽ ὅλον τὸ σῶμα. ὅταν

δὲ μὴ εὐπνοῆι τὸ σῶμα, νόσοι γίνονται, καὶ

διαφόρως· καθ᾽ ὅλον μὲν γὰρ τὸ σῶμα

50   τῆς ἀναπνοῆς ἐπεχομένης, νόσος

XXI   . . αθ . . . .

. . . σα . . . . τὰς γινομένας

. . . λλ . . . . κεινεῖσθαι

. . . μὴ . . . . εν τὰ ἠρε-

XX. 24.   αὐτονοεῖ or αὐτογνωμονεῖ.

XX views more peculiar to himself, saying that it is produced as the result of diseases. For whereas the others say that diseases come from bile, he says that bile comes from diseases. This thinker is in virtual agreement with Philolaus, in that he thinks that bile in us is merely useless. In this respect he agreed with Philolaus, in all other respects he has views of his own.

24 Philistion thinks that we are composed of four "forms," that is, of four elements—fire, air, water, earth. Each of these too has its own power; of fire the power is the hot, of air it is the cold, of water the moist, and of earth the dry. * * According to him diseases occur in many ways, but speaking quite generally and in outline we may call them three: (1) because of the elements; (2) because of the condition of our bodies; (3) because of external causes. * The elements cause disease when the hot and the moist are in excess, or when the hot becomes less and weak. * * External causes are of three kinds: (1) wounds and sores; or (2) excess of heat, cold and so on, or change of heat to cold, or of cold to heat; or (3) of nutriment to what is unsuitable or corrupt. * The condition of the body is a cause of disease in the following way. When, he says, the whole body breathes well and the breath passes through unhindered, health is the result. For breathing takes place not only by way of mouth and nostrils, but also over all the body. When the body does not breathe well, diseases occur, and in different ways. For when breathing is checked over all the body a disease . . . .

XXI. 25 . . . .

XXI 5 μοῦντα................τοντα

...ντ...................η ἐν τοῖς

..ασ...................ειλοντα

...εν σ..................ὡς νόσοι γίνονται

..εν ταῦτα............. * ἡμῖν δὲ

10 .δηκαιαν...........ἀνθρώπου ᾱ καὶ

...οι..............ασεως ταυ-

τη. δια...ηναπ...... παθῶν αἰτιο-

λογίας * συνέστηκεν δὲ ὁ ἄνθρωπος

ἐκ ψυχῆς καὶ σώματος. ὡς δ᾽ εἰς τοῦτο ὑπο-

15 τυπώσεως οὐ χρεία ἐστίν, περὶ μὲν ψυχῆς

ἄλλοις ἀναβάλλομαι· ἡμῖν δὲ τοῦ σώμα-

τος μελητέον, ἐπεὶ μάλιστα περὶ τοῦτο

σπουδάζει ἡ ἰατρική. * * τοῦ σώματος

μὲν οὖν τὰ μέν ἐστιν ἁπλᾶ μέρη, τὰ δὲ σύνθετα.

20 ἁπλᾶ δὲ καὶ σύνθετα λαμβάνομεν πρὸς αἴσ-

θησιν, καθὼς καὶ Ἡρόφιλος ἐπισημειοῦ-

ται λέγων οὕτως· "λεγέσθω δὲ τὰ φαινόμενα

πρῶτα, καὶ εἰ μὴ ἔστιν πρῶτα." ὁ μὲν γὰρ Ἐρασί-

στρατος καὶ πόρρω τοῦ ἰατρικοῦ κανό-

25 νος προῆλθε· ὑπέλαβεν γὰρ τὰ πρῶτα

σώματα λόγωι θεωρητὰ εἶναι, ὥστε τὴν

αἰσθητὴν φλέβα συνεστάναι ἐγ λόγωι

θεωρητῶν σωμάτων, φλεβός, ἀρτηρίας, νεύρου.

ἀλλὰ τοῦτον παραιτητέον. * ἡμῖν δὲ

30 λεκτέον, ὡς τῶν σωμάτων τὰ μὲν εἶναι ἁπλᾶ

τὰ δὲ σύνθετα, πρὸς αἴσθησιν τούτων λαμ-

βανομένων. * * ἁπλᾶ μὲν οὖν ἐστιν τὰ ὁμοιο-

μερῆ τὰ κατὰ τὰς τομὰς διαιρούμενα

εἰς ὅμοια μέρη ὡς ἐγκέφαλός τε καὶ νεῦ-

35 ρον καὶ ἀρτηρία καὶ φλὲψ καὶ τὰ ὑγρά.

28; cf. XXII. 51. Galen, XIV. 697 K.: καὶ Ἐρασίστρατος ὡς ἀρχὰς
καὶ στοιχεῖα ὅλου σώματος ὑποτιθέμενος τὴν τριπλοκίαν τῶν ἀγγείων
νεῦρα καὶ φλέβας καὶ ἀρτηρίας. Galen, II. 96 K.: φλέβας ἔχειν ἐν ἑαυτῷ
καὶ ἀρτηρίας τὸ νεῦρον ὥσπερ τινὰ σειρὰν ἐκ τριῶν ἱμάντων διαφερόντων
τῇ φύσει πεπλεγμένην.

---

10. The general sense is ἤδη καὶ ἀνάγκη εἰπεῖν περὶ ἀνθρώπου
πρῶτον καὶ ἐν τοῖς ἑξῆς ἀπὸ τῆς συστάσεως ταύτης διασημῆναι τὰς τῶν
παθῶν αἰτιολογίας. Cf. XXII. 5 (D.).

XXI   [It is now also necessary to speak about man first, and to go on from

this organism to make plain the aetiology of its affections.] Man is com-

posed of soul and body. And as there is no need to touch on it, I leave

the discussion of the soul to others; but we must pay attention to the

body, since medicine is chiefly concerned herewith. * *

26   Now some of the parts of the body are simple, and some are com-

pound. By "simple" and "compound" we mean what appear so to

our senses, following the terminology of Herophilus: "Let those things

be called primary that appear to be primary, even though they are not

really so." For Erasistratus went far beyond the medical rule when he

supposed that the primary bodies are observed only by reason, so

that the perceived vein is composed of bodies observed only by reason,

namely, vein, artery and sinew. We must beg to differ, * and assert

that of our bodies some parts are simple and some are compound, as

these are observed by our senses. * * Now things simple are of like

parts, that is, such as are by cutting divided into like parts, for example,

brain, sinew, artery, vein and the moist parts. For each of these is

14–16. The writer is uninterested in philosophy, including psychology.
See p. 27.

24. The ἰατρικὸς κανών means perhaps the standard adopted by
physicians generally. It may, however, refer to a body of accepted doctrine, independent of the vagaries of the schools, which furnished rules or
standards universally recognised. Cf. "canonical scriptures".

XXI   ἔκαστον γὰρ τούτων καὶ ὁμοιομερές ἐστιν
        καὶ τεμνόμενον εἰς ὅμοια χωρίζεται
        μέρη. * * σύνθετα δ' ἐστὶν τὰ ἀνομοιομερῆ ἢ τὰ
        κατὰ τὰς τομὰς εἰς ἀνόμοια χωριζό-
40   μενα μέρη ὡς χείρ, σκέλος, κεφαλή,
        ἧπαρ, πνεύμων, ἔκαστον τῶν τοιούτων·
        καὶ γὰρ ἀνομοιομερῆ ἐστιν καὶ κατὰ τὰς τομὰς
        εἰς ἀνόμοια χωρίζεται μέρη. * * τῶν δ' ἁπλῶν
        τὰ μέν ἐστιν κεκερματισμένα, τὰ δὲ ἡνωμένα.
45   κεκερματισμένα μὲν οὖν ἐστιν αἷμα, χολή, φλέ-
        γμα καὶ ὅλως πάντα τὰ ἐν ἡμῖν ὑγρά,
        ὁμοίως φῦσα, πνεῦμα, τὰ τούτοις ἐοικότα,
        ἡνωμένα δὲ τὰ μὴ τοιαῦτα. * * τῶν δὲ
        ἡνωμένων αὐτῶν τὰ μέν ἐστιν διατεταμέ-
50   να, τὰ δὲ παχέα τε καὶ διεστηριχότα,
        τὰ δὲ οὔτε διεστηριχότα οὔτε
        διατεταμένα. * * διατεταμένα μὲν οὖν
        νεῦρον, ἀδήν, ἀρτηρία, φλέψ, τὰ τούτοις

XXII   ἐγγύς. * * διεστηριχότα δὲ ὀστέα, χόν-
        δροι, τὰ ὅμοια. * τὰ μεταξὺ δὲ τούτων ἐνκέ-
        φαλος, μυελός, τὰ ἐοικότα· καὶ ἡ μὲν τοῦ
        ζώιου σύστασις ὡς ἐν κεφαλαίοις
5   τοιαύτη ἐστίν. * * ἰδίαι δὲ περὶ τῆς
        οἰκονομίας αὐτῆς νῦν ἀναγκαῖον δοκεῖ
        εἰπεῖν· οὕτως γὰρ ἂν εἴη σύμμετρον τῶι λόγωι·
        ἀπὸ πάσης δὴ τοίνυν τῆς συστάσεως τῶν
        σωμάτων συνεχεῖς μὲν ἀποφοραὶ γίνονται,
10   καὶ ἀπὸ τῆς ἐμψύχου μᾶλλον ἢ ἀπὸ τῆς
        ἀψύχου διά τε τὴν θερμασίαν καὶ
        διὰ τὴν κείνησιν, * ὅτι κατὰ τὴν διαφορὰν
        τῶν εἰρημένων ἀπὸ τῆς ἐν ἡμῖν θερμασίας
        μᾶλλον ἀποφοραὶ τῶν σωμάτων γίνονται ἢ ἀπὸ
15   τῶν ἐκτός· τὰ γὰρ ἑψόμενα καὶ ἁπλῶς θερ-
        μαινόμενα τῶν ὑδάτων μικρότερα γίνεται παρὰ
        τὴν θερμασίαν. .... τῶι ἄνω πνέου-
        σαν αὐτὴν φύσει συναποφέρειν ἑαυτῆι
        ἀτμοειδῶς πολλὴν ὑγρότητα καὶ ἅμα

XXII. 17.   Perhaps supply διὰ τί.

XXI both of like parts, and when cut up divides into like parts. * * Compound are those parts that are not homogeneous, that is, those that on cutting divide into unlike parts, such as hand, leg, head, liver, lung, and each such-like part. These in fact are not homogeneous, and on cutting divide into unlike parts. * * Of the simple parts, some are finely divided while others are united. Now the finely divided are blood, bile, phlegm, and in general all the moist things in us, with gas and breath, and things like these. United parts are such as are not like these. * * Of the united parts themselves some are extended, others stout and firm, others neither firm nor extended. * * Now extended XXII are sinew, gland, artery, vein and the like. * * Firm are bones, cartilages and similar parts. * Between these come the brain, marrow and things like them. Such in general is the structure of animals. * * It now appears necessary to speak particularly about its maintenance, for this would be appropriate to our discussion. Well then, from all the structure of a body come continuous emanations, more from a living structure than from a lifeless, on account of the warmth and the movement, * because, corresponding to the difference between the aforesaid parts, emanations from our bodies occur more, because of the warmth in us, than from external objects. For water when boiled, or simply heated, becomes less because of the warmth......Warmth, naturally wafted upwards, with itself bears away much moisture in the form of

---

XXI. 47. Probably φῦσα in this sentence is air generated in the body, "gas"; πνεῦμα is what we breathe.

XXII. 6. It is impossible to keep the same English word for οἰκονομία in the passage that follows.

XXII 20 λεπτυνόμενον ὑπ᾽ αὐτῆς τὸ ὑγρὸν
ἀτμοειδῶς ἀποφέρεσθαι. καὶ οὕτως μὲν
ἐπὶ τῶν ἐκτός. διὰ ταὐτὰ δὲ δοκεῖ γίνεσθαι ἡ
ἀποφορὰ πρὸς τῆς θερμασίας ἐπὶ τῶν
ἡμετέρων σωμάτων. * ἠτμισμένα γὰρ..
25 δύναται ἀποφέρειν ταυτ.των. καὶ τὰ μὲν βαρέα
καὶ παχέα δυσκόλως διαφορεῖται, τὰ δὲ
κοῦφα καὶ ἐλαφρὰ εὐχερῶς, ὡς ἂν δὴ
τῆς κεινήσεως αἰτίας ὑπαρχούσης τῆς ἀποφορᾶς.
καὶ γὰρ τὸ μὲν κατεραμμένον ἔδαφος
30 οὐ πάνυ πολλὴν ἀποφορὰν ποιεῖται
διὰ τὸ βάρος, τὸ δὲ κατάξηρον πλείστην
διὰ τὴν κουφότητα, ᾗ καὶ κονιορτὸς
ἀποφέρεται πολύς, ἅτε δὴ τῆς κεινήσεως
παραιτίας τούτων ὑπαρχούσης. διὰ τὴν κείνησιν
35 οὖν ὡς ὁμοίως ἀποφορὰ ἀπὸ τῶν σωμάτων
γίνεται συνεχής. * τούτων δὴ οὕτως ἐχόντων
καὶ ἀποφορᾶς συνεχοῦς γινομένης
ἀπὸ τῶν ἡμετέρων σωμάτων, εἴπερ ἀντὶ τῶν ἀποφερομένων μὴ ἐγείνετο εἰς τὰ
40 σώματα πρόσθεσις, κἂν διεφθείρετο ῥαιδίως
τὰ σώματα. * ὅθεν ἡ φύσις ἐμηχανήσατο
ὀρέξεις τε τοῖς ζώιοις καὶ ὕλην καὶ δυνάμεις, * ὀρέξεις μὲν εἰς τὸ τὴν ὕλην αἱ-
ρεῖσθαι, * ὕλην δὲ εἰς ἀναπλήρωσιν τῶν ἀπο-
45 φερομένων, * δυνάμεις μέντοι γε εἰς διοί-
κησιν τῆς ὕλης· καὶ γὰρ οὐδὲν ὄφελος ἦν
ὀρέξεως, εἰ μὴ ὕλη παρῆν. οὐδὲ μὴν
ὕλης ὄφελος ἦν, εἰ μὴ δυνάμεις παρῆ-
σαν αἱ διοικονομοῦσαι. * * ἀλλὰ γὰρ ὕλην
50 ὑπεβάλετο τροφήν τε καὶ πνεῦμα·
δύο γὰρ πρῶτα καὶ κυριώτατά ἐστιν, οἷς διοι-

---

51. Galen (XIV. 697) gives a different account of Erasistratus, saying
that he made blood nutriment, breath a συνεργὸν εἰς τὰς φυσικὰς ἐνεργείας,
but neither an ἀρχή.

---

25. Read ταῦτα ἀπ᾽ αὐτῶν.
28. D. suggests παραιτίας, comparing l. 34.
51, 52. ἀεὶ δεῖται K.

XXII steam, and at the same time the liquid, thinned out by it, is evaporated
in the form of steam. This is what happens on external bodies. For
the same reasons, it is thought, the emanation takes place on our own
bodies because of the warmth. * For warmth can evaporate from
bodies these particles when reduced to steam. Heavy, thick particles
are thrown off with difficulty, the light and active particles easily,
as would be so when motion is the cause of the emanation. Just as a
besprinkled floor sends up very little cloud because of the weight,
but a parched floor sends up very much, because of the lightness,
whereby much dust is carried away, inasmuch as the motion is a
contributory cause of these things. So in a like way it is motion that
makes the emanation from bodies to go on continuously. * These things
therefore being so, and evaporation occurring continuously from our
bodies, if in place of the evaporating matter there were not occurring
additional supplies to our bodies, these bodies would easily perish. *
Wherefore nature designed for animals appetites, material and
powers—appetites for the taking of material, * material to replace
what is evaporated, * and powers for the assimilation of the material.
For were not material present, appetite would be of no use, nor
would material be of use were not powers present which assimilate
it. * * But, in fact, nature laid a material foundation of nutriment
and breath. For these are two primary essentials, by which, as

23. ἐπί might mean "in the case of", as Cornford would prefer.
27. ὡς ἂν δή: used to introduce a fact in accordance with, or the
cause of, one just mentioned; "as would be so", "as is natural because",
"consistent with the fact that". See XXIV. 37, XXV. 8, 14, 52, XXXIV. 1,
XXXV. 5.

XXII κεῖται τὸ ζῷον, ὥς φησιν ὁ Ἐρασίστρατος.
ἔνιοι δὲ ἐνκαλοῦσιν αὐτῶι καὶ λέγουσιν ἐκεῖνο ᾱ· οὐ μόνον δύο εἶναι

XXIII ....
..........κυριώτατα· ὑπερβολὴν γὰρ οὐ-
δετέρου ἡμῖν εἶναι ἀναγκαίαν. γ̄· οὐδὲ τούτοις πρώτοις διοικονομεῖται τὸ ζῷον, ἀλλὰ αὐτά ἐστιν
5 διοικονομούμενα ὑπὸ τῶν δυνάμεων.
καὶ ταῦτα μὲν λέγουσι πρὸς τὸν Ἐρασίστρατον,
ἃ ὕστερον ἐν οἰκείωι τόπωι πρὸς ἡμῶν δια-
πορηθήσεται. * * ἐπεὶ δὲ ὕλην ὑποβέβληται
τοιαύτην αἴτια τιθεὶς τροφήν τε καὶ πνεῦμα
10 ἁπάντων, περὶ τῆς ἑκατέρου διοικήσεως
λαλήσομεν, καὶ πρότερον περὶ τῆς τοῦ πνεύματος·
ἕλκεται τοιγάρτοι τὸ πνεῦμα ἔξωθεν
ὑπὸ τοῦ στόματος καὶ τῶν μυκτήρων
καὶ διὰ τῆς τραχείας ἀρτηρίας φέρεται εἰς
15 πνεύμονα καὶ καρδίαν, ἔτι δὲ θώρακα·
διηθεῖται δὲ καὶ εἰς κοιλίαν ὀλίγον διὰ τοῦ
στομάχου καθ᾽ ἡμᾶς, * οὐ μὴν δὲ κατὰ
τὸν Ἐρασίστρατον. * * ἀπὸ τούτων δὴ τῶν τόπων
φέρεται εἰς τὰς κατὰ μέρος ἀρτηρίας. φέρεται
20 δὲ καὶ εἰς τὰ κοιλώματα· ὡς ὁμοίως δὲ
καὶ εἰς τὰ καθ᾽ ὅλον τὸ σῶμα ἀραιώματα,
εἶτα διεκθεῖ διὰ τῶν ἐν τῆι σαρκὶ φυσικῶν ἀραιωμάτων εἰς τὸ ἐκτός. τὸ δὲ πλεῖον ἐκπνεῖται διά τε τοῦ στόματος καὶ τῶν μυκτή-
25 ρων. * * καὶ δὴ τοῦ εἰσπνεομένου πλεῖον
ἐκπνεῖται διὰ τούτων τῶν τόπων, λέγω δὲ διὰ
στόματος καὶ μυκτήρων, ὅπερ ἐστὶν ἴσως παράδοξον. πῶς γὰρ οἷόν τ᾽ ἐστὶν πλεῖον ἐκπνεῖσθαι,

---

XXIII. 11. Cf. Galen, IV. 466 K.: ἀρχὴ μὲν οὖν διὰ τοῦ στόματος καὶ
τῶν ῥινῶν ἑλκόμενος ἀὴρ ὕλη τυγχάνων τῆς κατὰ τὴν ἀναπνοὴν χρείας...
διὰ τῆς τραχείας ἀρτηρίας εἰς τὸν πνεύμονα κομιζόμενος.

XXIII. 1, 2. The sense requires τὰ πρῶτα, ἀλλὰ πλείω. β̄· οὐδὲ ταῦτα
εἶναι τοῖς σώμασι κυριώτατα. (D.)

XXII Erasistratus says, an animal is maintained. But some criticise him thus: (1) there are not only two primaries, but more; (2) nor are these XXIII essential for our bodies, for excess of neither is a necessity for us; (3) again, they are not primaries by which an animal is maintained, but they are themselves maintained by the powers. This is what they say in reply to Erasistratus, which later at the appropriate place will be the subject of enquiry before us. * * Since he regards such material as fundamental, postulating nutriment and breath as the causes of all things, we shall speak about the maintenance of each, and firstly about that of breath. Accordingly breath is inhaled by the mouth and nostrils, and is carried through the wind-pipe to the lungs and heart, and further to the trunk. A little too filters through to the belly through the mouth of the stomach, as we maintain, * contrary however to Erasistratus. * * Now from these places it is borne into the branch arteries. It is also borne into the cavities. Similarly also into the pores throughout the whole body, and then it percolates through the natural pores in our flesh to the outside. The greater part is exhaled through the mouth and nostrils. * * And furthermore there is exhaled through these places, I mean through the mouth and nostrils, more breath than is inhaled—which may appear absurd. For how is it possible for more

XXIII. 2, 3.   Two possible meanings in Greek as in English: (1) absence of excess is a necessity; (2) there is no need of any excess.

5.   Nutriment and breath might be said to be maintained or administered by the powers of the body so that full use can be made of them.

7.   This promise is not fulfilled.

9. and 11.   For πνεῦμα see p. 10. Here perhaps "spirit".

15.   θώρακα: ἀπ' αὐχένος μέχρι αἰδοίων, Aristotle, H.A. I. 7, 1.

21.   The word ἀραιώματα was apparently used by some physiologists instead of πόροι.

XXIII καίτοι γε ἀπὸ τοῦ εἰσπνεομένου ἀναλου-
30   μένου τινὸς εἰς τὰ σώματα; ἀλλ' οὐκ ἔστιν πα-
      ράδοξον· ὃν γὰρ τρόπον κατατάσσεταί τι εἰς
      τὰ σώματα ἀπὸ τοῦ εἰσπνεομένου, τὸν
      αὐτὸν τρόπον καὶ τῶι πνεύματί τινα προστί-
      θεται ἀπὸ τῶν σωμάτων καὶ πλείονά γε, ἅτινα
35   καὶ πλεῖον ἀποτελεῖ τὸ ἐκπεμπόμενον
      πνεῦμα. * * ψυχρόν τε ὑπάρχον τὸ πνεῦμα
      θερμὸν ἐκπέμπεται, ἅτε δὴ φερόμενον
      διὰ σωμάτων θερμῶν. ἀμέλει γὰρ τὴν
      εἰσπνοὴν γίνεσθαί φησιν εἰς τὸ τὸ πλεῖον θερμὸν
40   τὸ περὶ τὴν καρδίαν καταζβέννυσθαι καὶ
      μὴ σωματούμενον καταφλέγειν τὰ σώ-
      ματα. * * τούς τε ὕπνους, ὥς φησιν ὁ Ἀριστοτέλης,
      ἀποτελεῖσθαι τοῦτον τὸν τρόπον· τῆς
      γὰρ καρδίας φύσει θερμῆς ὑπαρχούσης
45   καὶ ἐξ αὐτῆς ἀνηρτημένου τοῦ θερμοῦ,
      τοῦ δ' ἐνκεφάλου ψυχροῦ, συμβέβηκεν
      περὶ τῶι ἐνκεφάλωι συνίστασθαι
      ὑγρότητα τὴν ἀναφερομένην ὑπὸ
      τῆς θερμότητος ἀπὸ καρδίας,

---

42. Aristotle, de somno et vigilia, 3 (456a 30–32): ἐχόμενον δὲ
τῶν εἰρημένων ἐστὶν ἐπελθεῖν, τίνων γινομένων καὶ πόθεν ἡ ἀρχὴ τοῦ
πάθους γίγνεται, τοῦ τ' ἐγρηγορέναι καὶ τοῦ καθεύδειν. Ibidem (456b
17–24): οὐκ ἔστιν ὁ ὕπνος ἀδυναμία πᾶσα τοῦ αἰσθητικοῦ, ἀλλ' ἐκ τῆς
περὶ τὴν τροφὴν ἀναθυμιάσεως γίνεται τὸ πάθος τοῦτο· ἀναγκαῖον γὰρ τὸ
ἀναθυμιώμενον μέχρι του ὠθεῖσθαι, εἶτ' ἀντιστρέφειν καὶ μεταβάλλειν
καθάπερ εὔριπον, τὸ δὲ θερμὸν ἑκάστου τῶν ζώων πρὸς τὸ ἄνω πέφυκε
φέρεσθαι· ὅταν δ' ἐν τοῖς ἄνω τόποις γένηται, ἀθρόον πάλιν ἀντιστρέφει
καὶ καταφέρεται. Ibidem (456b 26–28): ὅταν δὲ ῥέψῃ κάτω καὶ ἀντιστρέψαν
ἀπώσῃ τὸ θερμόν, τότε γίνεται ὁ ὕπνος καὶ τὸ ζῶον καθεύδει. Ibidem
(457b 29, 30): πάντων δ' ἐστὶ τῶν ἐν τῷ σώματι ψυχρότατον ὁ ἐγκέφαλος,
τοῖς δὲ μὴ ἔχουσι τὸ ἀνάλογον τούτῳ μόριον. Ibidem (458a 1–5): οὕτως
ἐν τῇ ἀναφορᾷ τοῦ θερμοῦ τῇ πρὸς τὸν ἐγκέφαλον ἡ μὲν περιττωματικὴ
ἀναθυμίασις εἰς φλέγμα συνέρχεται (διὸ καὶ οἱ κατάρροι φαίνονται γιγνό-
μενοι ἐκ τῆς κεφαλῆς), ἡ δὲ τρόφιμος καὶ μὴ νοσώδης καταφέρεται
συνισταμένη καὶ καταψύχει τὸ θερμόν. Ibidem (458a 8–12): τῆς μὲν οὖν
καταψύξεως τοῦτ' ἐστιν αἴτιον, καίπερ τῆς ἀναθυμιάσεως ὑπερβαλλούσης
τῇ θερμότητι, ἐγείρεται δ', ὅταν πεφθῇ καὶ κρατήσῃ ἡ συνεωσμένη
θερμότης ἐν ὀλίγῳ πολλὴ ἐκ τοῦ περιεστῶτος.

XXIII to be exhaled, when moreover some part of the inhaled breath is expended on our bodies? However it is not absurd. For just as a part of the inhaled breath is assigned to our bodies, even so to the breath certain additions are made, and these too greater than the amount lost, which make the exhaled breath actually greater than the inhaled. * * The breath, cold to begin with, is exhaled warm, inasmuch as it is borne through warm bodies. Of course the inhaling takes place, he says, with a view to reducing the excessive heat about the heart, and to prevent its becoming solid and burning up our bodies. * * And sleep, as Aristotle says, is brought about in this way. The heart is by nature hot, and on it heat depends, while the brain is cold, the consequence being that there gathers about the brain moisture brought up

34. καὶ πλείονά γε: perhaps, "very considerable".

38–42. There were two views current in antiquity about the function of breathing: (1) that breath cooled the "innate heat" about the heart; (2) that breath produced heat by combustion with corporeal elements. See Clifford Allbutt, *Greek Medicine at Rome*, pp. 224–264. From Galen (IV. 471) we learn that view (1) was held by Philistion and Diocles, but that Erasistratus thought that we breathe ἐπιπληρώσεως ἕνεκεν ἀρτηριῶν. This makes φησιν (XXIII. 39) difficult to understand.

42. As we see from the *Testimonia* Aristotle explained sleep as the result of a flow of heat from the brain to the heart, whereby the brain is cooled.

XXIII 50 ἦν δὴ συνισταμένην καταψύχεσθαι
καὶ ἐκ τοῦ . . . . πάλιν καταφέρεσθαι,
μὴ δυναμένην διὰ τὸ ψῦχος διαμέ-
νειν ἐν τοῖς τόποις, ἐπὶ τὴν καρδίαν

XXIV . . . .
καὶ τῆι μίξει τὸ θερμόν. * ὧδε τὸν ὕπνον γίνεσθαι,
τὴν δὲ ἐγρήγορσιν ἀποτελεῖσθαι ἀναλουμένης
τῆς ὑγρότητος ἁπάσης τῆς περὶ τῶι ἐγκεφάλωι,
5 ἔπειτα τοῦ θερμοῦ πάνυ πλεονάζοντος. καίτοι γε ἑαυτὸν ἐπαινεῖ ὁ Ἀριστοτέλης, ὅτι παρὰ τοὺς
ἄλλους καὶ τὸν ὕπνον καὶ τὴν ἐγρήγορσιν αἰτιο-
λογεῖ ἐκείνων αὐτὸν μόνον τὸν ὕπνον αἰτιο-
λογούντων, μηκέτι δὲ καὶ τὴν ἐγρήγορσιν.
10 πλὴν περὶ οὗ ὁ λόγος, τὸ πνεῦμα ψυχρὸν εἰσπνεῖται,
θερμὸν μέντοι γε ἐκπνεῖται, ὡς δὴ διὰ θερμῶν
χωρίων φερόμενον. * καὶ μὴν ξηρὸν μὲν εἰσπνεῖται, ὑγρὸν δὲ ἐκπνεῖται· καὶ δῆλον· *
εἰ γάρ τις περὶ τοῦ στόματος καὶ τοῦ μυκτῆρος
15 τὴν χεῖρα ἢ μέρος τοῦ ἱματίου προθείη,
συνόψεται ἔνικμον τοῦτο, ὡς δὴ σὺν
τῶι πνεύματι καὶ ὑγρότητος συνεκπεμπο-
μένης. καὶ περὶ μὲν τῆς τοῦ πνεύματος διοικήσεως ταῦτα. * * περὶ δὲ τῆς τροφῆς ἀναγ-
20 καῖον ὑπομιμνήσκειν μετὰ ταῦτα· αὕτη προσενεχθεῖσα
πρώτης κατεργασίας τυγχάνει ἐν στόματι
τεμνομένη μὲν πρὸς τῶν προσθίων ὀδόν-
των — τομεῖς καλοῦνται —, καταλεαινομέ-
νη δὲ πρὸς τῶν μυλῶν, λοιπὸν καταπείνεται
25 διὰ στομάχου καὶ φέρεται εἰς κοιλίαν.
κἂν ταύτηι δὲ μεταβάλλει τε καὶ ἀποικειοῦται
χυλουμένη ἐπὶ τὸ οἰκεῖον. καὶ γὰρ ἀρέσκει
ἡμεῖν τὴν τροφὴν ἐν κοιλίαι μεταβάλλειν
τε ἐπὶ τὸ οἰκεῖον κἂν ταύτηι δευτέρας κατερ-

XXIV. 6.   Not to be found in Aristotle.

XXIII. 51.   In the gap K. detects κατα. This, as D. suggests, may
represent κατάρρου or ἐνκεφάλου.
XXIV. 14.   For the περὶ of P. we should probably read πρό.

XXIII from the heart by the heat, which gathers, cools and sinks again out

of the . . . . . . .not being able, because of the cold, to remain in these

XXIV places, to the heart. . . . . .and by the mixing, heat. * In this way sleep

takes place, while waking occurs when the heat is in great abundance

because the moisture about the brain is being all expended. And yet

Aristotle praises himself because he, in contrast to the others, gives

the reason for both sleep and waking, whereas they give the reason

for sleep only, not for waking. However, to go back to our subject,

breath is inhaled cold but exhaled hot, as it passes through places

that are hot. * Furthermore, it is dry when inhaled, but moist when

exhaled. Here is proof. * If you put your hand, or a part of your

cloak, in front of the mouth and nostrils, you will see at a glance that

this is humid, showing that moisture also is sent out with the breath.

27   So much for the maintenance of the breath. * * Next we must make

some mention of nutriment. This when taken undergoes a first stage of

digestion in the mouth, being cut up by the front teeth, called incisors,

and ground by the molars. Finally it is swallowed down the gullet,

and is carried to the belly. And in this it changes, becoming juice and

assimilating itself to that which is akin to it. In fact it is our opinion

that nutriment changes in the belly to that which is akin, and in the

XXIII. 51.   Add perhaps "brain".
XXIV. 6.   From no extant work of Aristotle.
9.   For μηκέτι see p. 33.
14.   The conjecture πρό is translated.

XXIV 30 γασίας τυγχάνειν καὶ οὐχ ὥσπερ ὁ Ἀσκληπιάδης ὁ οἰνοδώτης καὶ Ἀλέξανδρος
ὁ Φιλαλήθειος διέλαβον, ὡς τέμνεται μόνον
καὶ χυλοῦται ἡ τροφὴ ἐν κοιλίαι καὶ προδιάθε-
σίς τις αὐτῆι γίνεται, †ου μην† οὐ μὴν ἀποικείωσις
35 ἐπὶ τὸ οἰκεῖον. * * ἡμεῖς γὰρ λέγομεν καὶ χυλοῦσθαι
τὴν τροφὴν ἐν κοιλίαι καὶ κατεργασίας τυγχάνειν καὶ μεταβολῆς
τῆς
ἐπὶ τὸ οἰκεῖον, ὡς ἂν δὴ διὰ τούτων καὶ θερ-
μοτέρων παραφερομένην χωρίων· καὶ
δεόντως ὥσπερ κἀπὶ τῶν ὑδάτων· ταῦτα
40 γὰρ ῥέοντα διά τινων τόπων μετα-
λαμβάνει τῆς ἀπ᾽ ἐκείνων δυνάμεως
καὶ τὴν αὐτὴν κείνοις ἴσχει δύναμιν.
ἐὰν γὰρ ὦσιν οἱ τόποι ἀσφαλτώδεις, καὶ
τὸ ὕδωρ ἀσφαλτῶδες γίνεται κατὰ τὴν δύναμιν,
45 ἐὰν δὲ θειώδεις, θειώδη μεταβάλλον-
τα γίνεται καὶ τὰ ὕδατα. ὡς οὖν ταῦτα μεταβάλλει τὰς δυνάμεις παρὰ τὰς τῶν τόπων
διαφοράς, οὕτως κἀπὶ τῆς τροφῆς· αὕτη γὰρ .... θερ-

---

30. Pliny, *H.N.* XXIII. 38: *Asclepiades utilitatem vini aequari vix deorum potentia posse pronuntiavit.* Idem, XXVI. 14: *trahebat* (Asclepiades) *praeterea mentis artificio animos iam vinum promittendo aegris dandoque tempestive, iam frigidam aquam. et quoniam causas morborum scrutari prius Herophilus instituerat, vini rationem inlustraverat Cleophantus apud priscos, ipse cognominari se frigida danda praeferens, ut auctor est M. Varro, alia quoque blandimenta excogitabat.* Idem, VII. 124: *Asclepiadi Prusiensi condita nova secta spretis legatis et pollicitationibus Mithridatis regis reperta ratione qua vinum aegris mederetur, relato e funere homine et conservato* etc. Apuleius, *Florida,* 19, p. 32, 14 Krüger: *Asclepiades ille inter praecipuos medicorum, si unum Hippocratem excipias, ceteris princeps primus etiam vino repperit aegris opitulari, sed dando scilicet in tempore.* Caelius Aurelianus, *acut. morb.* II. 39 (Amman, p. 175): *iubet etiam dari vinum noctibus diurnis atque iugiter, sed id vinum cui salem admiscuerimus et quod appellavit* τεθαλασσωμένον *...probat autem vinum dandum post cibum, siquidem solum facile penetret ac pertranseat corpora non aliter quam si sine ulla faece per liquatoria fundatur... iubet etiam meracum, non mixtum dari. hac enim ratione, inquit, exustae viae tanquam ex igni conductae sudorem retinendo constringunt.*

---

31. οινοδωτης P.

XXIV belly undergoes a second stage of digestion, differing in this from Asclepiades the wine-giver and Alexander Truth-lover, who supposed that in the belly nutriment is only cut up and reduced to juice, and that what happens to it is a sort of predisposition, and not assimilation to that which is akin. * * For we say that nutriment is both reduced to juice in the belly and also undergoes a process of digestion and change to that which is akin, seeing that it is carried along through these and warmer regions. This is what must happen, as it does also in the case of water. For water, when it flows through certain places, partakes of their property and acquires the same property as they have. For if the places be bituminous, the water too becomes bituminous in character; if they be sulphurous, the water too changes and becomes sulphurous. So as water changes its properties to correspond to the various qualities of the places, so it is also in the case of nutriment . . . .

30, 31.   For Asclepiades and Alexander see p. 14.
37.   Or, "these and yet warmer". It is difficult to see whether καὶ means *hoc est* or whether it adds something fresh.
39.   δεόντως: either "should" or "must", probably the second.
41.   For δύναμις see p. 9. Here "characteristic" and (44) "character" might serve.
47.   παρὰ is perhaps merely "because of".

XXIV 50 μοτέρων τόπων.................. νην
ἐν κοιλίαι καὶ .... χυς τόποι μὲν ἢ τ..................εται
τῶι ....ροι πο
λωνον και .... κατερ-

XXV γασίας τυγχάνει. * ἀναλαμβανομένη δὲ
πρὸς τῶν ἀγγείων τῶν ἀπὸ τοῦ μεσεντερίου μὲν
ἐκφυόντων, ἐνφυόντων δὲ εἰς τὴν κοιλίαν
προστίθεται τῶι ὅλωι σώματι * καὶ μὴν
5 καὶ ἀτμοειδῶς διὰ τῶν ἀραιωμάτων
τῶν ἐν τῆι κοιλίαι ἀναλαμβάνεται ἡ τροφὴ
καὶ ἐξ ὠμῶν γίνεται ἡ πρόσθεσις τῶι ὅλωι σώματι,
ὡς ἂν δὴ καὶ ἐξ ὠμῶν γινομένης τῆς
ἀναδόσεως. καὶ ἐν τῶι στόματι δὲ ληφθεί-
10 σης τῆς τροφῆς παρὰ ταῦτα ἀνάδοσις γίνεται ἀπ' αὐτῆς, ὡς ἂν δὴ πάλιν καὶ ἐξ ὠμῶν γινομένης
τῆς ἀναδόσεως. ταύτηι δὴ καὶ οἱ κατάξηρα
ἴσχοντες τὰ στόματα διακλυσάμενοι
μαλακώτερα φέρονται, ὡς ἂν δὴ ἀναδόσεως
15 παραυτὰ γινομένης. * ἀμέλει δὲ τούτωι
τῶι λόγωι καὶ δυσώδη προσφερόμενοι διωθούμεθα
αὐτὰ κατὰ τὴν παραυτὰ γενομένην
γεῦσιν, καὶ ἐκδ ὧν ἀντιλαμβανόμεθα καὶ αὐτὰ δῆ[λα].
ἐξ ὧν φανερόν, ὡς καὶ ἐξ ὠμῶν γίνεται ἡ ἀνάδοσις.
20 ἀλλὰ γὰρ καὶ κατὰ τὴν κατάποσιν τὴν διὰ στομάχου
τῆς τροφῆς ἀνάδοσις γίνεται καὶ πρόσθεσις τῶι ὅλωι.
ἐξ ὧν φανερόν, ὡς καὶ πέψις γίνεται καὶ ἐν κοιλίαι,
καὶ ἐξ ὠμῶν δὲ ἡ ἀνάδοσις. ταύτηι δὴ
καὶ τοῦ Ἀσκληπιάδου διοίσομεν· οὗτος γὰρ
25 ἐξ ὠμῶν αὐτὸ μόνον λέγει γίνεσθαι τὴν ἀνάδοσιν,

XXV. 25. [Galen], *Defin. med.* 99 (XIX. 373): οἱ δὲ ἐξ ὠμῶν ἔφασαν τὰς
ἀναδόσεις γίγνεσθαι, ὥσπερ καὶ Ἀσκληπιάδης ὁ Βιθυνός. Caelius Aurelian.
ac. morb. I. 14 (p. 44 Amman): *neque ullam digestionem in nobis esse, sed
solutionem ciborum in ventre fieri crudam et per singulas particulas corporis ire,
ut per omnes tenuis visa penetrare videatur quod appellavit* λεπτομερές
(cf. Galen, IV. 706 f.), *sed nos intelligimus spiritum.*

XXV. 10. παραυτὰ H. Schöne.
17. Perhaps γινομένην.
18. P. has δη only; D. reads δῆλα.

XXIV ....

XXV ....undergoes a process of digestion. * And being taken up by the vessels that grow out of the mesentery and into the belly it is added to the whole body. * Furthermore nutriment is absorbed also in the form of vapour through the pores in the belly, and also the addition to the whole body comes from crude foods, since from crude foods too absorption may take place. And in the mouth, too, when nutriment has been taken, because of these things absorption takes place from it, conformably again with the view that absorption occurs even from crude foods. In just this way too, also, those who have dry mouths, after a wash-out, are eased, implying that absorption at once takes place. * This of course is the reason why on putting into our mouth things with a disagreeable savour we reject them on the strength of the taste that immediately arose, and from the sensations we receive the things themselves also are recognised. Whence it is clear that from crude foods also absorption occurs. But as a matter of fact absorption of nutriment and addition to the whole body occurs also by way of swallowing through the gullet. Whence it is clear that in addition to the digestion that takes place in the belly there is also absorption from crude foods. In this respect we shall be found also to differ from Asclepiades. For he says that this—I mean absorption—takes

XXV. 9 ff. It is not clear whether these instances are given to prove that crude foods are absorbed, or as examples only, the absorption being assumed. From l. 19 it seems that the former alternative is more natural.

18. "Und auch aus dem, was wir annehmen, ist es ebenfalls klar": B. and S. The fact that we recognise at once the true character of nauseous things as soon as we put them into our mouth shows that some absorption takes place there. We might have expected for δυσώδη a more general term meaning "nasty", but taste and smell are closely allied. D. says that ἐκδ = ἐξ, but surely Hackforth's suggestion ἐκ δ' is right.

XXV ἡμεῖς δὲ καὶ ἐξ ὠμῶν μὲν καὶ ἐκ πέψεως
τῆς ἐν κοιλίαι γινομένης. * καὶ τοῦ Ἐρασιστράτου δὲ
διοίσομεν, καθ' ὅσον κεῖνος μὲν τὸ μὲν αἷμα εἶπεν
μόνον εἶναι τροφήν, ἡμεῖς δὲ καὶ τὸ αἷμα μὲν
30 εἶναι τροφήν, μὴ μόνον δέ, ἀλλὰ καὶ τὴν ὠμὴν
δὲ τροφήν. * * εἶτα τῆς τροφῆς ἡ μὲν εὔχυμος
καὶ λεπτομερεστέρα αὐτόθεν ἀναδίδοται τῶι
ὅλωι σώματι διαχωροῦσα, ἡ δὲ στερεὰ καὶ τραχεῖα πέσσεται
ἐν κοιλίαι· πέψις γάρ ἐστιν μεταβολὴ κ.......ις ἐπὶ τοι..ι
35 σαι· διαίρεσις γάρ. * καὶ οὐ μόνον ἐν κοιλίαι
36a–c γίνεται ἀνάδοσις, ἀλλὰ πάσης τῆς τροφῆς ἄπεπτόν τι λείπε | ται
καὶ φέρεται εἰς τὰ ἔντερα καὶ ἐν τούτοις | ἀναδίδοται, καὶ ἐν
τοῖς ἐντέροις οὐκ αὐτοῖς —
ἡ γὰρ μερισθεῖσα εἰς ταῦτα τροφὴ ἀναδίδοται
ἢ διὰ τῶν περὶ αὐτὰ ἀραιωμάτων ἢ διὰ τῶν ἀγγείων
τῶν ἐμφυόντων εἰς αὐτά — καὶ οὐ πᾶσα, ἐλάχιστον
40 δὲ ταύτης ἀπολείπεται, ὃ δὴ πρὸς τῆς ἐν τῶι
κόλωι ἰδιότητος ἀποκοπροῦται. γίνεται δὲ καί τι τοῦ
σπέρματος. καὶ γὰρ τοῦτο κατασκευάζεται
πρὸς τῆς ἰδιότητος τῆς ἐν τοῖς σπερματικοῖς
πόροις μεταβαλλούσης τὴν φερομένην
45 ὡς αὐτοὺς τροφήν. οὕτως δὴ καὶ τὸ διαλλάττον
πρὸς τῆς ἐν ἑκάστωι ἰδιότητος γίνεται .... τροφή ἐστιν
ἐν τοῖς ἐντέροις ἔξω μεγίσ-
θ
των οὕτως ἐχόντων ἕτερον κατ....ν
καὶ ἀπὸ τῶν ἐντέρων ἀνάληψις γίνεται
τῆς τροφῆς. τὸ μὲν γὰρ ἐν τῶι λεπτῶι ἐντέρωι
50 παρακείμενον λεπτότερόν τ' ἐστὶν καὶ
ὑγρότερον, τὸ δὲ ἐν τῶι ἀπευθυσμένωι
ξηρότερον καὶ παχύτερον, ὡς ἂν δὴ
πρὸς τούτων ἀναδόσεως γεγενημένης.
αὐτὰ δὲ τὰ ἀποκρινόμενα περισσώματα τροφὴ

---

27. Galen, II. 112 K.: ἐπὶ δὲ τῆς τοῦ αἵματος γενέσεως οὐδὲν ἀτιμο-
τέρας οὔσης τῆς ἐν τῇ γαστρὶ χυλώσεως τῶν σιτίων οὔτ' ἀντειπεῖν τινι
τῶν πρεσβυτέρων ἠξίωσεν οὔτ' αὐτὸς εἰσηγήσασθαί τινα ἑτέραν γνώμην
ἐτόλμησεν (Erasistratus).

---

34. λείωσις ἐπὶ τὸ ἑψῆσαι D., comparing Galen, XIX. 372.
36a–c restored from writing between the lines and in the margin.
46. Perhaps μία γὰρ ἡ τροφή ἐστιν ἐν τοῖς ἐντέροις.

XXV place from crude foods only, whereas our contention is that it occurs both from crude foods and from the digestion that takes place in the belly. * And we shall be found to differ from Erasistratus also, in so far as he said that the blood alone is nutriment, but we say that the blood, while being nutriment, is not the only one, as there is also crude nutriment. * * Then, too, the part of nutriment that is juicy and composed of smaller particles is absorbed straight away by the whole body during its passage through it, while the part that is hard and rough is digested in the belly. For digestion is a change and grinding fine as an aid to seething, being a kind of division. * And not only in the belly does absorption take place, but of all the nutriment a part is left undigested and is carried into the intestines, and in these is absorbed, but not actually in the intestines; for the nutriment dispersed into them is absorbed either through the pores around them or through the vessels that grow into them; and not all of it, as a very small part of it is left, which passes out as excrement owing to the peculiar characteristic of the colon. A part of it too is added to the seed. This in fact is brought about by the peculiar characteristic in the spermatic passages that changes the nutriment brought to them. It is even so, by the peculiar characteristic in each part, that the various changes occur . . . . . . is the food in the intestines . . . . this being so one thing . . . . . . and the absorption of food takes place also from the intestines. For that which lies along the small intestine is smaller and moister, while that in the straight intestine is drier and coarser, implying that absorption has taken place through their action. The residues themselves that are excreted become the nutriment of others, nutri-

41. "It becomes also something of the seed."
42. τοῦτο may refer to τι or to σπέρμα.
46 ff. It is hopeless to attempt a restoration of this passage, which must, however, have contained instances of food becoming one constituent or another of the body, according to the δυνάμεις or ἰδιότητες of the passages along which it travels.
50. The force of παρα- in this compound, here as in XXVIII. 34, seems to be "along". In other passages, e.g. XXXVI. ·38, XIV. 21 and 25, it means "near", "alongside".

XXVI ἄλλων γίνεται, τροφὴ δὲ τῶν ἀλόγων ζῴων. * πρὸς τοῦτο τὰ μὲν περισσώματα τροφή ἐστιν τῶν ἀλόγων
ζώιων, αὕτη δὲ πρὸς αὐτῶν λαμβανομένη
μεταβάλλει εἰς τὴν σάρκα. * οὕτω καὶ αὐτῶν
5 γίνεται τροφή, εἰς μέντοι γε τὰς τῶν ἀλόγων ζώιων
σάρκας προσφερόμενα οἷον ὀρνείθων καὶ τῶν
παραπλησίων, καὶ πρὸς τούτων τρεφόμεθά τε
καὶ αὐξανόμεθα. τῶι δὲ αὐτῶι λόγωι τροφή
ἐστιν αὖ τῶν ἀνθρώπων τὰ περισσώματα. *
10 εἰ δεῖ οὖν τροφὴν εἶναι τῶν ἀνθρώπων τὰ περισσώματα,
ἐπειδὴ τὰ ἄλογα τῶν ζώιων τρέφεται πρὸς
τῶν περισσωμάτων καὶ αὔξεται, ἡμεῖς δὲ
πρὸς τῶν ἀλόγων ζώιων, τούτωι τῶι λόγωι
φησὶν καὶ τὸ ξύλον καὶ τὸν λίθον καὶ
15 τὰ παραπλήσια τροφὴν εἶναι, ἐπειδὴ πάντα εἰς πάντα μεταβάλλει. ἄλογον δὲ τοῦτο. * διὰ τί γὰρ τὰ θανάσιμα
τῶν . . . . ν κα. . ευου. . επι. τροφή, εἴπερ οἱ οἴσυπος . . ουν . . . οι τὸ κώνειον τρέφουσι
τοὺς ἀνθρώπους; * πλὴν ταῦτα μὲν οὕτως.
20 ἐκεῖνο δὲ ῥητέον, ὅτι γίνεται καὶ ἐν κοιλίαι πέψις
καὶ εὐχύμων δὲ ἀνάδοσις, * ἡ πλείων
δὲ ἀνάδοσις ἀπό τε κοιλίας καὶ στομάχου
καὶ ἀπὸ τῶν ἐντέρων καὶ τοῦ κόλου — καὶ
γίνεται ἡ ἀνάδοσις διὰ τῶν ἀραιωμάτων τῶν ἀμφ᾽ αὐτά —
25 καὶ ἀπὸ τοῦ στόματος. καὶ οὐ μόνον ἀπὸ
τούτων ἀνάδοσις γίνεται καὶ πρόσθεσις, ἀλλὰ καὶ
ἀπὸ τῶν ἐν τοῖς ἀγγείοις παρακειμένων
καὶ ἀπὸ τῆς ἐν ταῖς φλεψὶν παρακει-
μένης τροφῆς· καὶ ἀπὸ τῆς ἐν ταῖς ἀρ-
30 τηρίαις ἀνάδοσις γίνεται καὶ πρόσθεσις τῶι ὅλωι

---

4. Cornford suggests αὐτῶν ⟨τῶν ανων⟩ or αὖ τῶν ⟨ανων⟩.
17. D. says "desperandus locus". He adds, referring to Galen, XII.
309, "ergo sensus esse videtur: si omnia mutentur alia ex aliis, nos
omnia eodem modo nutriant τὸ πεπτικὸν οἴσυπος ὁμοίως καὶ τὸ θανάσιμον
κώνειον."

XXVI ment, that is, of the irrational animals. * Therefore the residues are the nutriment of the irrational animals, and this taken in by them changes into their flesh. * So they become nutriment for men too; it is however by being added to the flesh of the irrational creatures, e.g. of birds and the like, and by these we are nourished and grow. By the same reasoning the residues of men become once more their nutriment. * If therefore the residues of men must be their nutriment, since the irrational animals are nourished and grow by the residues, and we by the irrational animals, on this reasoning, he says, both wood and stone and suchlike things are nutriment, since all things turn into all things. But this argument is absurd. * For why are deadly poisons not nutriment, if men are nourished as much by hemlock as by the digestive suint? * Be this as it may, we must state that in the belly too there takes place digestion, with absorption of juicy substances; * but the greater part of the absorption is from the belly and gullet, and from the intestines and the colon (and the absorption takes place through the pores that are about these parts), and also from the mouth. And not only from these do absorption and addition take place, but also from what lies along the vessels, and from the nutriment that lies along the veins. Absorption also takes place from the nutriment in the arteries, with addition to the whole body,

4. Perhaps αὐτῶν = τῶν ἀλόγων ζῴων, as otherwise ll. 8, 9 merely repeat what has been said already (Hackforth). But Anonymus retains the lecturer's repetitions.
14. Query, Erasistratus?
17, 18. Though the text is mutilated the sense is plain.
21. The argument is far from clear.
27. For παρακειμένων see p. 99.

XXVI   σώματι καὶ ἀτμοειδῶς. * ὁ μέντοι γε Ἐρασίστρα-

τος οὐκ οἴεται ἀνάδοσιν γίνεσθαι ἀπὸ τῶν ἀρτηριῶν.

μὴ γὰρ εἶναι κατὰ φύσιν ἐν αὐταῖς αἷμα — τοῦτό ἐστιν

τροφή —, ἀλλὰ πνεῦμα, οὐχ ὑγιῶς ἱστάμενος λόγον,

35   ὡς ἀποδείξομεν. εἷς μὲν γάρ· εἴπερ μὴ παρέκει-

το ἐν ἀρτηρίαις κατὰ φύσιν αἷμα, ἐχρῆν

διαιρουμένων ἀρτηριῶν αἷμα μὴ ἀποκρίνεσθαι·

ἀποκρίνεται μέντοι, ὥστε γίνεται τροφὴ ἐν ταύταις.

πρὸς ὃν λόγον ἀπολογοῦνται οἱ Ἐρασιστρά-

40   τειοι λέγοντες, διότι διαιρέσεως γενομένης

κατὰ τὰς ἀρτηρίας κενοῦται τὸ αἷμα κἀπορεῖ

τῶν ἐκεῖ φλεβῶν, οὐ μὴν ἐκ τῶν ἀρτηριῶν.

διαφέρει δὲ τὸ διά τινος κενοῦσθαι ἢ τὸ

ἐκ τούτου καὶ ἐπὶ τῶν ἐκτός. καὶ γὰρ διὰ τῶν

45   κρουνῶν ῥεῖν φαμεν ὕδωρ, οὐ μὴν ἐκ τῶν κρουνῶν·

οὕτω δὲ καὶ τῶν ἀρτηριῶν διαιρεθεισῶν

δι' αὐτῶν μὲν κενοῦται τὸ αἷμα, οὐ μὴν ἐξ αὐ-

---

31. Galen, III. 492 K.: ὅσοι ταῖς ἀρτηρίαις οὐδ' ὅλως αἵματος μετα-
διδόασιν ὥσπερ καὶ ὁ Ἐρασίστρατος. Idem, II. 104 K.: εἰ δὲ τὴν διὰ τῶν
φλεβῶν φορὰν τῆς τροφῆς ἀνάδοσιν καλεῖ (Erasistratus), τὴν δ' εἰς ἕκαστον
τῶν ἁπλῶν καὶ ἀοράτων ἐκείνων νεύρων καὶ ἀρτηριῶν μετάληψιν οὐκ
ἀνάδοσιν ἀλλὰ διάδοσιν, ὥς τινες ὀνομάζειν ἠξίωσαν. Ibidem (p. 95 K.):
εἰ δ' ἐπισκοποῖτό τις ἐπιμελῶς, οὐδ' ὁ περὶ θρέψεως αὐτοῦ λόγος, ὃν ἐν
τῷ δευτέρῳ τῶν καθόλου λόγων διεξέρχεται (Erasistratus), τὰς αὐτὰς
ἀπορίας ἐκφεύγει. τῇ γὰρ πρὸς τὸ κενούμενον ἀκολουθίᾳ συγχωρηθέντος
ἑνὸς λήμματος, ὡς πρόσθεν ἐδείκνυμεν, ἐπέρανέ τι περὶ φλεβῶν μόνων
καὶ τοῦ κατ' αὐτὰς αἵματος. ἐκρέοντος γάρ τινος κατὰ τὰ στόματ' αὐτῶν
καὶ διαφορουμένου καὶ μήθ' ἀθρόου τόπου κενοῦ δυναμένου γενέσθαι μήτε
τῶν φλεβῶν συμπεσεῖν... ἀναγκαῖον ἦν ἕπεσθαι τὸ συνεχὲς ἀναπληροῦν
τοῦ κενουμένου τὴν βάσιν.

XXVI and in the form of vapour. * Erasistratus however does not think that absorption takes place from the arteries. For he says that there is not naturally in them blood (that is nutriment), but breath, putting forward, as we shall show, an unsound argument. Here is one point. Suppose blood did not naturally lie along the arteries, then, when arteries were severed, it would be necessary for blood not to flow from them. However, it does so flow, so that in them nourishing does take place. The followers of Erasistratus reply to this argument that, when a cutting has been made in the arteries, the blood empties itself and flows from the veins thereby, but does not flow out of the arteries. But there is a difference between an emptying "through" a thing and an emptying "out of" it, which difference can be seen also in things outside the body. For in fact we say that water flows "through" its well-heads, but not "out of" its well-heads. So too when the arteries have been severed, the blood is emptied through them, but not out of them. For they

31. Apparently from 16 to 31 the author is giving his own opinions, turning here once more to refute Erasistratus.

33. According to Erasistratus only blood is nutriment. See XXV. 28. For μὴ see p. 33.

34 (and 48d). For πνεῦμα, here perhaps "air", see p. 10.

35. With εἰς understand λόγος.

43. "Through", when the place through which was merely a passage, not the place of origin (ἐκ).

XXVI τῶν· οὐ γὰρ εἶναι λέγουσιν ἐν ταύταις αἷμα. τότε γὰρ | συνε-
στομῶσθαί τε τὰς φλέβας εἰς τὰς ἀρτηρίας καὶ | τὸ ἐνὸν
48 a οὕτωι μὴ δύνασθαι κενὸν ἀθροῦν ἀπολείπεσθαι τόπον μετὰ
| τὴν πνεύματος κένωσιν. παρεμπείπτειν | γὰρ τὸ αἷμα ἐκ τῶν
48 g φλεβῶν εἰς τὰς ἀρτηρίας· | διὰ μέντοι τῶν ἀρτηριῶν ἀπορεῖν
ἐκ τούτων ὡς | διὰ καλάμων ἔξω.
νωθρὸν δέ ἐστιν λείαν τοῦτο * ἃ μὲν γὰρ τὰ ἡμέ-
50 τερα σώματα τοῖς ἀσυμπτώτοις ἔοι-
κε σώμασιν ὡς σίφωσί τε καὶ καλάμοις· ὡς
γὰρ οὗτοι καταχθέντες ἢ τρυπηθέντες οὐκ ἀποκρίνου-

XXVII σι τὸ ἐν αὐτοῖς περιεχόμενον πνεῦμα
οὐδὲ κενοὶ γίνονται τούτου, ἀλλ᾽ ἐμμένον ἔχουσιν
ἐν αὐτοῖς, οὕτως καὶ ἐπὶ τῶν ἀρτηριῶν διαιρεθεισῶν
οὐ πάντως κενωθήσεται τὰ [ἐντὸς] τοῦ πνεύματος,
5 ἀλλ᾽ ἐμμενεῖ ἐν ταῖς ἀρτηρίαις καὶ μετὰ τὴν

XXVI. 48. Galen, XI. 152 K.: ἄριστα οὖν μοι δοκῶ διαθέσθαι τὸν λόγον,
εἰ τἆλλα παραλιπὼν ἀπ᾽ αὐτῶν ἀρξαίμην τῶν Ἐρασιστράτῳ δοκούντων...
ἀρέσκει δ᾽ αὐτῷ πνεύματος μὲν ἀγγεῖον εἶναι τὴν ἀρτηρίαν, αἵματος δὲ
τὴν φλέβα· σχιζόμενα δ᾽ ἀεὶ τὰ μείζω τῶν ἀγγείων εἰς ἐλάττονα μὲν τὸ
μέγεθος, ἀριθμὸν δὲ πλείω καὶ πάντη τοῦ σώματος ἐνεχθέντα (μηδένα
γὰρ εἶναι τόπον, ἔνθα μὴ πέρας ἀγγείου κείμενον ὑπάρχει) εἰς οὕτω
σμικρὰ πέρατα τελευτᾶν, ὥστε τῇ μύσει τῶν ἐσχάτων στομάτων κρατού-
μενον ἐντὸς αὐτῶν ἴσχεσθαι τὸ αἷμα· καὶ διὰ τοῦτο καίτοι παρακειμένων
ἀλλήλοις τοῦ στόματος τοῦ τε τῆς φλεβὸς καὶ τῆς ἀρτηρίας, ἐν τοῖς ἰδίοις
ὅροις μένειν τὸ αἷμα μηδαμόθι τοῖς τοῦ πνεύματος ἐπεμβαῖνον ἀγγείοις.
μέχρι μὲν δὴ τοῦδε νόμῳ φύσεως διοικεῖσθαι τὸ ζῷον· ἐπεὶ δέ τις αἰτία
βίαιος ἐκ τῶν φλεβῶν εἰς τὰς ἀρτηρίας τὸ αἷμα μεταχθῆναι, αὐτὸ νοσεῖν
ἀναγκαῖον ἤδη. Idem, IV. 709: καὶ διὰ τοῦτ᾽ ἐξ ἀνάγκης ἕπεται τὸ διὰ
τῶν συναναστομώσεων, ὡς αὐτός φησιν, αἷμα τῇ πρὸς τὸ κενούμενον
ἀκολουθίᾳ, καὶ τοῦθ᾽ ὥσπερ προδεδεμένον τῷ κατὰ τὰ πέρατα τῶν
ὑστάτων ἀρτηριῶν πνεύματι, πρῶτον μὲν ἅπαντος τοῦ ἄλλου αἵματος,
ὕστατον δὲ παντὸς τοῦ κατὰ τὰς ἀρτηρίας πνεύματος κενωθήσεται.
XXVI. 48 f. (cf. 51). Galen, II. 75 K.: ἐπὶ μὲν γὰρ τῶν καλάμων καὶ
τῶν αὐλίσκων τῶν εἰς τὸ ὕδωρ καθιεμένων ἀληθὲς εἰπεῖν, ὅτι κενουμένου
τοῦ περιεχομένου κατὰ τὴν εὐρυχωρίαν αὐτῶν ἀέρος ἢ κενὸς ἀθρόος ἔσται
τόπος ἢ ἀκολουθήσει τὸ συνεχές, ἐπὶ δὲ τῶν φλεβῶν οὐκέτ᾽ ἐγχωρεῖ
δυναμένου δὴ τοῦ χιτῶνος αὐτῶν εἰς ἑαυτὸν συνιζάνειν καὶ διὰ τοῦτο
καταπίπτειν εἰς τὴν ἐντὸς εὐρυχωρίαν. οὕτω μὲν δὴ ψευδὴς ἡ περὶ τῆς
πρὸς τὸ κενόμενον ἀκολουθίας οὐκ ἀπόδειξις μὰ Δί᾽ εἴποιμ᾽ ἄν, ἀλλ᾽
ὑπόθεσις Ἐρασιστράτειος.

XXVI. 48 a ff. The extra lines are written in the margin and on the bottom.

XXVI say that there is no blood in them; for when the veins, which are joined by a mouth to the arteries, are cut, the inside, after the emptying of the air, cannot be left a continuous vacuum. For the blood trickles in out of the veins into the arteries. So it flows through the arteries from the veins outwards as through reeds. But this is a very feeble explanation. * For in the first place our bodies are like bodies that are not likely to collapse, such as pipes and reeds. For just as these XXVII when broken or pierced do not let the air escape that is confined in them, and do not become empty of it, but keep it remaining in them, even so in the case of the severed arteries the insides will not be entirely emptied of air, but it will remain in the arteries even after the severing,

XXVI. 48a. The subject is the followers of Erasistratus. For μὴ see p. 33.

48c, d. By κενὸς ἀθρόος τόπος is meant a considerable void, not just enough to permit of movements of atoms. See note D, p. 12.

XXVII διαίρεσιν, ὥσπερ κἀπὶ τῶν ἐκτός · * * β · εἴπερ ὁ κενὸς
ἀθροῦς αἴτιος γίνεται τῆς παρεμπτώσεως τοῦ αἵματος
ἐκ τῶν φλεβῶν εἰς τὰς ἀρτηρίας, ἀνάγκη τὸν
αὐτὸν αἴτιον γίνεσθαι τῆς κατοχῆς τοῦ πνεύματος, οὕτως τὸ
θ
αἴτιον . . . . ω
10 ἀλλὰ γὰρ οὐ γίνεται· ὥστε τὸ αἴτιον παρορᾶν δεῖ. * * ναί,
φασὶν οἱ Ἐρασιστράτειοι, οὐκ ἔοικε
τὰ ἡμέτερα σώματα τοῖς ἀσυμπτώτοις
σώμασιν, ἃ κυρίως κατωνόμασται, ἀλλὰ ἀσκῶι
ἐνπεπληρωμένωι ὑγροῦ καὶ ἐμπεπνευμα-
τωμένωι ωσο.νον, ὃς τρωθεὶς ἀποκρείνει
15 δι᾽ αὐτοῦ τό τε πνεῦμα καὶ ὑγρόν, ἅμα δὲ καὶ
ἐξ ἑαυτοῦ· οὕτως καὶ αἱ ἀρτηρίαι διαιρεθεῖσαι
αἷμα, οὐκ ἐξ αὐτῶν δέ· * πρὸς δὲ καὶ τοῦτ᾽ εἴποιμεν, διότι οὐ τοῖς οὖσι συμπτώτοις ἔοικεν
τὰ ἡμέτερα σώματα, ὥς φασιν πταίοντες,
20 ἀλλὰ τοῖς ὑπάρχουσιν ἀσυμπτώτοις, ὡς ταῦτα
δῆλα ἐπὶ τῶν τελευτῶν· κατὰ γὰρ τὰ ὑμένια
εὑρίσκονται αἱ ἀρτηρίαι ἀσύμπτωτοι, ἀλλ᾽ οὗτοι σύμπτωτοι.
εἰ τοιγάρτοι ταῦτα τοῦτον ἔχει τὸν τρόπον,
μοχθηροὶ φαίνονται καὶ κατὰ ταῦτα οἱ Ἐρασιστράτειοι.
25 εἶτα φέρε δὲ καὶ οἰκειοῦντες μὴ τοῖς
ἀσυμπτώτοις, ἀλλὰ τοῖς εὐσυμπτώτοις
ὡς ἀσκοῖς, ἵνα καὶ αὐτοῖς συναγορεύω-
μεν, λέγωμεν, ὡς ἐπὶ τοῦ ἀσκ[οῦ τοῦ ἐνόντος κενωθέντος
ἐπισύμπτωσις γίνεται, καὶ οὐχὶ κενὸς ἀθροῦς τόπος]. ἀλλὰ
ἐχρῆν καὶ ἐπὶ τῆς διαιρέ-
30 σεως τῶν ἀρτηριῶν μετὰ τὴν κένωσιν
τοῦ πνεύματος ἐπισυμπείπτειν ταύτας.
ἐπισυμπειπτουσῶν δὲ αὐτῶν οὐκ ἂν ἐγίνετο
κενὸς ἀθροῦς οὐδὲ παρέμπτωσις αἵματος
οὐδὲ ἀπόκρισις τούτου οὐδέ γε κένωσις·
35 ὥστε καὶ κατὰ ταῦτα αγαν . . . ις. * * φέρε
δὲ μετὰ τὴν διαίρεσιν εὐθὺς ἀποκρινομένου
τοῦ πνεύματος εἴπωμεν εἰσκρίνεσθαι

9b. D. suggests αὐτῷ ἂν ἐναντιωθείη.
14. Perhaps ὡς οἴνου.
21. Perhaps τετελευτηκότων.
35. The sense requires something like ἄγαν νωθεῖς.

XXVII just as in the case of external objects. * * Secondly, if the continuous vacuum is the cause of the irruption of blood from the veins into the arteries, the same must be the cause of the retention of the air. Thus the argument contradicts itself. But in fact it is not the cause of it. So that we must reject this explanation. * * Yes, say the followers of Erasistratus, our bodies are not like uncollapsible bodies, properly so called, but like a bladder filled with liquid and inflated, which on being pierced lets escape through itself, and at the same time out of itself, both the air and liquid. So too the arteries, when severed, let blood escape through, but not out of themselves. * In reply to this also we would say that our bodies are not like collapsible things, as they erroneously assert, but such as are uncollapsible, as is shown when people are dead. For then the thin walls of the arteries are found uncollapsible, and not at all collapsible. Therefore, if this be the case, the followers of Erasistratus in this respect also show themselves to be poor scientists. Come then, comparing the arteries, not to uncollapsible things, but to things easily collapsible, such as bladders, in order that we may agree with this sect, let us say that, in the case of the bladder, when its content has been emptied a collapse takes place and not a continuous vacuum. But on the severing of the arteries also there should have taken place a collapse of them after the emptying of the air. And on the collapse of them there would not occur a continuous vacuum, nor an irruption of blood, nor a secretion of it, nor yet an emptying of it. So in this respect also the Erasistrateans prove very stupid. * * Now then, let us say that, the air being let out immediately after the severing, the

9b. I translate D.'s suggested supplement.

14. The suggested supplement would mean "e.g. with wine". A similar experiment in [Hippocrates], *Nature of the Child*, xxv: L. VII. 522.

17. εἴποιμεν: perhaps we should change to εἴπωμεν, or ἄν may have been lost after -εν. It may be potential without ἄν, a common construction in the Hippocratic *Corpus*.

19. The subject is the followers of Erasistratus.

XXVII

    τὸ αἷμα τῶι μὴ τόπον κενὸν ἀθροῦν
    ἀπολειφθῆναι. ἀλλὰ μὴν οὐκ ἐχρῆν αἷμα
40 κενοῦσθαι τούτωι τῶι λόγωι, ἀλλὰ τὸ πνεῦ-
    μα τὸ ἐν τῆι ἡμετέραι παρακείμενον
    συγκρίσει λείως συναφίεσθαι τῶι πνεύματι
    τῶι ἀποκριθέντι. οὐκ ἀποκρίνεται δέ
    γε τοῦτο καὶ συνπληροῖ τὸν τοῦ κενωθέντος
45 πνεύματος τόπον . . . .
    εἶτα κατὰ τοὺς Ἐρασιστρατείους τούσδε ὅ-
    τε κενοῦται μενον καὶ λ . . . . . αἷμα . . . . .
    Ἐρασιστράτειοι . . ει . . . . . αι διαδοῦναι
    τῶν ἐπι . . . . τοῦ
50 πνεύματος . . . πολ . . . . του . . .
    †παραδητας† τοτ . . . . σδε τω . .
    πρώτη †θη† κενώσεται . . . .
    κατατοῦ μεταιονᾶι οσ . . . . κε-

XXVIII

    νωθῆναι τὸ ἐν ταῖς ἀρτηρίαις τῶι πο-
    λὺ κεχωρίσθαι ταύτας τῆς καρδίας.
    καὶ πάλι πρώτη πληρωθήσεται αἵματος πρὸς τῶν φλεβῶν,
    οὕτως τε πολὺς χρόνος γενήσεται,
5   ὥστε μετὰ τὴν κένωσιν τοῦ πνεύματος
    ῥυῆναι τούτων τὸ αἷμα. * * καὶ ἐπὶ πᾶσιν, εἴ-
    περ ἡ καρδία πρώτη κενουμένη τοῦ πνεύματος
    πρώτη καὶ πληροῦται κατὰ τὴν παρέμπτωσιν
    αἵματος, λέγω ἀναιρεθήσεται τὸ ζῷον τῶι ἐν ἀνοι-
10 κείωι γίνεσθαι τόπωι τὸ αἷμα καὶ δεσπόζοντι τοῦ ζώιου μέρει.
    οὐκ ἔχει δὲ ταῦτα
    τοῦτον τὸν τρόπον. πολλῶν γὰρ διαιρουμένων ἀρτηριῶν οὐδὲν
    ἀπέθανεν· οὐκ ἄρα ὑγιής ἐστιν ἡ τῶνδε τῶν
    Ἐρασιστρατείων κεκομψευμένη δόξα. * * τούτων
    οὕτως ἐκκειμένων, ὅτι μὲν καὶ διὰ τὰς †ωτ† ἀρτηρίας ἐστὶν
    ἀνάδοσις, ὑπεμνήσαμεν· ὅτι δὲ καὶ κατὰ τὰς
15 ἀρτηρίας †τηριων† προαπεδείξαμεν. καὶ πλείων γε

XXVII. 53. "μεταιοναι clare P." (D.).
XXVIII. 9. P. has clearly λέγω, but D. conjectures λόγῳ, as contrasted
with ἔργῳ δὲ οὐκ ἀναιρεῖται. Perhaps παρέμπτωσιν, αἵματος λέγω,
(Hackforth).
   13. The sense requires φλέβας for ἀρτηρίας.
   15. I suggest προσαπεδείξαμεν.

XXVII blood is let in because a continuous vacuum has not been left. But in truth on this reasoning blood should not have been emptied, but the air that is present throughout our physical frame should have been gently discharged along with the let-out air. But this is not let out, and fills up the space left by the emptied air. . . . . . . Then according to these Erasistrateans . . . .

. . . .

XXVIII the air in the arteries to be expelled because these are far separated from the heart. And again, it will be the first to be filled with blood by the veins, and so much time will elapse, so that it is after the expulsion of the air that the blood flows from these. * * and in all cases since the heart, being the first to be emptied of the air, is also the first to be filled by the irruption of blood, the animal will be destroyed, I say, by the blood's getting in an unsuitable place, and in a part which is supreme over the animal. But these things are not so. For many arteries can be cut without any death at all. So the neatly worked out idea of these Erasistrateans is not sound. * * These facts having been set forth, we mentioned that through the veins also there is absorption; we have further shown that it also takes place along the arteries. And in the veins

XXVIII. 13–16. The text is very much disturbed in this passage, the transcriber's attention having apparently wandered. See critical note. There is no point in distinguishing διὰ τὰς ἀρτηρίας from κατὰ τὰς ἀρτηρίας, φλέβας for the former ἀρτηρίας being almost certainly correct. I suggest too that προσαπεδείξαμεν be read for προαπεδείξαμεν. It is difficult to decide whether the mistakes are due to the note-taker or to the transcriber.

XXVIII   ἡ ἐν ταῖς †απο των† φλεψὶ †βων† ἀνάδοσις ἥπερ ἐν ταῖς †απο
των† ἀρ-
τηρίαις †ων†, ὡς ἀποδείξομεν. ᾱ μὲν γὰρ ἀξιολογώ-
τεραί εἰσιν αἱ φλέβες τῶν ἀρτηριῶν· πιθανὸν δὲ
ἐν τῶι ἀξιολογωτέρωι πλείονα γίνεσθαι τὴν
20   ἀνάδοσιν παρὰ τὰ ἐλάχιστα ταῦτα.
ἀξιολογώτεραι δέ εἰσιν τῶν ἀρτηριῶν αἱ φλέβες,
ἐν αἷς εἰκότως πλείων γενήσεται ἡ ἀνάδο-
σις. β̄· καὶ εἰ ἴσαι εἰσὶν κατὰ τὸ μέγεθος αἱ ἀρτηρίαι
ταῖς φλεψίν — φέρε γὰρ οὕτως ἔχειν — εἰ δ' οὖν [ἴσαι,]
25   αἱ μὲν ἀρτηρίαι μείζονες οὖσαι κατὰ τὴν περιοχὴν αὐτὸ μόνον φανήσονται τῶι τε
τετραχίτωνες εἶναι καὶ συνεστάναι ἐξ εὐρώσ-
των τῶν χιτώνων. * αἱ δὲ φλέβες ἀσθενέσ-
τεραι ὑπάρχουσαι κατὰ τὴν περιοχὴν τῶι μονοχί-
30   τωνες εἶναι ὅμως εὐρυκοιλιώτεραί
εἰσιν τῶν ἀρτηριῶν, εὐρυκοιλιώτεραι δὲ
οὖσαι πλείονα ἕξουσιν καὶ τὴν ἀνάδο-
σιν τὴν εἰς αὐτὰς γινομένην. * * τὸ δὲ γ̄· αἱ μὲν ἀρτηρίαι πλεῖον ἔχουσι τὸ παρακείμενον ἐν αὐταῖς πνεῦμα,
35   ἐλάχιστον δὲ τὸ αἷμα, * αἱ.δὲ φλέβες πλεῖον
ἔχουσι τὸ αἷμα, ἐλάχιστον δὲ τὸ πνεῦμα.
ἀρέσκει γὰρ ἡμῖν καὶ ἐν ἀρτηρίαι καὶ ἐν φλεβὶ
κατὰ φύσιν παρακεῖσθαι καὶ αἷμα καὶ πνεῦμα,
οὕτως δὲ ταῦτα παρακεῖσθαι, κα-
40   θὼς πρόκειται. * πλὴν ἐπεὶ ἐν μὲν ἀρτηρίαι
†πλειον† πλεῖον τὸ πνεῦμα, ἐν δὲ φλεβὶ
ἐναντίον τοῦτο, πιθανώτερον πλείονα
γίνεσθαι ἐν φλεβὶ τὴν ἀνάδοσιν ἥπερ ἐν ἀρτηρίαι.
καὶ διὰ μὲν τούτων συνακτέον, ὡς πλείων
45   [γίνεται] ἡ ἀνάδοσις ἐκ τῶν φλεβῶν ἥπερ ἐξ ἀρτηριῶν.
ὁ μέντοι γε Ἡρόφιλος ἐναντίως διείλη-
φεν· οἴεται γὰρ πλείονα μὲν γίνεσθαι ἀνάδοσιν
ἐν ταῖς ἀρτηρίαις, * ἥσσονα δὲ ἐν
ταῖς φλεψὶ διὰ δύο ταῦτα· ᾱ μέν, ἐπει-
50   δήπερ ἀμφότεραι μὲν ὀρεκτικῶς ἔχουσι
τῆς τροφῆς, ἥ τε φλὲψ καὶ ἡ ἀρτη-

16. P. had originally ἡ ἀπὸ τῶν φλεβῶν ἀνάδοσις ἥπερ ἀπὸ τῶν
ἀρτηρίων.
20. ἐλάχιστα ταῦτα K.: "vix sensui apta" D.

XXVIII the absorption is greater than in the arteries, as we shall proceed to show. For in the first place the veins are more important than the arteries. And it is plausible that in the more important part the absorption taking place is greater in comparison with that in these very trivial parts. But more important than the arteries are the veins, in which the absorption will naturally prove to be greater. Secondly, even if the arteries are equal in size to the veins —assuming such to be the case—if then they are equal, the arteries will prove to be greater in circumference only because their coverings are fourfold, and because these coverings are very strong in texture. * Veins, though being weaker on their outer surface owing to their having one covering only, yet are of wider capacity than are the arteries, and being of wider capacity they will also allow a greater absorption to take place into them. * * Thirdly, the arteries have throughout their length more air but very little blood * while the veins have more blood but very little air. For the view that we support is that both blood and air normally are found along both artery and vein, and that they are found to occur in the way we have set forth. * Save that, since in an artery the air is the greater, while in a vein the reverse is the case, it is more probable that more absorption takes place in a vein than in an artery. For these reasons it must be inferred that absorption from veins is greater than from arteries.

28   Herophilus however has taken the opposite view. For he thinks that more absorption takes place in the arteries * and less in the veins for the two reasons that follow. First, since both crave nourishment, both

XXIX   ρία, ἐπεὶ δὲ κατ' ἴσον ὀρέγονται τῆς τροφῆς,
          κατ' ἴσον καὶ ἡ ἀνάδοσις εἰς αὐτὰς γενήσεται.
          δεύτερον δὲ αἱ μὲν ἀρτηρίαι, φησίν, συστέλλον-
          ταί τε καὶ διαστέλλονται τόν τε σφυγμὸν
5   ἀποδιδόασιν, αἱ δὲ φλέβες οὔτε συστέλλον-
          ται οὔτε διαστέλλονται οὐδὲ σφυγμωδῶς
          κεινοῦνται. * ἐπεὶ τοιγάρτοι αἱ μὲν ἀρτηρίαι
          σφυγμωδῶς κεινοῦνται, αἱ δὲ φλέβες
          οὐ κεινοῦνται σφυγμωδῶς, ταύτηι ἐπὶ τῶν
10   ἀρτηριῶν διὰ τὴν ὦσιν ἐκείνην εὔλογον πλείονα γίνεσθαι τὴν
          ἀνάδοσιν ἥπερ ἐπὶ τῶν φλεβῶν διὰ τὴν
          εἰρημένην αἰτίαν. * * οὐκ ὀρθῶς δὲ ὁ προκεί-
          μενος ἀνὴρ ἐποίησεν. οὐ γὰρ ἐνόησεν, ὡς
          εὐρυκοιλιώτεραί εἰσιν αἱ φλέβες παρὰ τὰς
15   ἀρτηρίας, εὐρυκοιλιώτεραι δὲ οὖσαι
          πλείονα δεόντως ἕξουσι καὶ τὴν ἐν αὐ-
          ταῖς γινομένην ἀνάδοσιν. καὶ πρὸς μὲν τὸ ᾱ
          τούτου κεφάλαιον τοῦτο καθήξει λέγειν,
          πρὸς δὲ τὸ δεύτερον ἐροῦμεν, διότι
20   αἱ ἀρτηρίαι σφυγμωδῶς κεινοῦνται συστελ-
          λόμεναι καὶ διαστελλόμεναι, οὕτως δὲ κεινού-
          μεναι ἐκθλείψουσιν εἰς τὸ ἐκτὸς τὴν τρο-
          φήν· εἰ δὲ ταῦτα οὕτως ἔχει, ὁμολογουμένως
          ἐπισυνάγεται, ὅτι πλείων ἀνάδοσις γίνεται τρο-
25   φῆς εἰς τὰς φλέβας ἥπερ εἰς τὰς ἀρτηρίας. * ἀλλὰ
          ὁμολογουμένως κἀκεῖνο δεῖ ὑπονοῆσαι, ὡς
          τροφὴ παράκειται ἐν ταῖς ἀραιότησι τῶν φλεβῶν
          καὶ τῶν ἀρτηριῶν. καὶ κοινῶς ἐν πάσηι ἀραιό-
          τητι τετμημένηι κατὰ τὸ ἡμέτερον σῶμα
30   παράκειται τροφή, καὶ ἀνάδοσις γίνεται εἰς αὐτὴν
          ὁμολογουμένως τῶι ὅλωι σώματι, ὥστε καὶ

---

3. Galen, VIII. 702 K.: ἔτι δὲ μείζων ἄλλη διαφορὰ τοῖς ἰατροῖς ἐκ
παλαιοῦ περὶ τῶν ἀρτηριῶν ἐγένετο τινῶν μὲν ἡγουμένων αὐτὰς ἐξ ἑαυτῶν
σφύζειν..., ἐνίων δὲ σφύζειν μὲν αὐτὰς [so Susemihl for αὐτοῦ] τοῦ
χιτῶνος αὐτῶν διαστελλομένου τε καὶ συστελλομένου, καθάπερ ἡ καρδία,
τὴν δύναμιν δ' οὐκ ἐχουσῶν σύμφυτον ἧ τοῦτο δρῶσιν, ἀλλὰ παρὰ καρδίας
[so H. Schöne for καρδίαν] λαμβανουσῶν· ἧς γνώμης ἔχεται καὶ Ἡρόφιλος.
Ibidem, VIII. 717: φαίνεται γὰρ ὁ ἀνὴρ οὗτος [Herophilus] ἅπασαν ἀρτηριῶν κίνησιν...ὀνομάζων σφυγμόν.

XXIX vein and artery, and since they crave it equally, equal also will be the absorption that takes place into them.   Secondly, the arteries, he says, contract and expand, so producing the pulse, while the veins neither contract nor expand, and produce no throbbing of the pulse. * Since therefore arteries produce a pulse-throbbing while the veins do not do so, therefore in the case of the arteries because of that pressure it is likely that for the reason given more absorption takes place than in the case of the veins. * * But the writer in question made a blunder. For he did not realise how the veins are of wider capacity as compared with the arteries, and being of wider capacity they will of necessity permit the absorption too that takes place in them to be greater. To the first main point of Herophilus it will be appropriate to make this reply; in answer to the second point we shall say that as the arteries produce a pulse by contracting and expanding, so by a pulsation they will squeeze out the nourishment to the outside. And if this be the case the incontestable inference is that there takes place greater absorption of nutriment into the veins than into the arteries. * But this too must be accepted as an incontestable truth, that nourishment is present throughout the pores both of the veins and of the arteries. And generally in every pore pierced throughout our body there is present nutriment, and absorption takes place into each pore incontestably for the whole

27. The force of παρα- in the compound seems to be "all along", "throughout". Possibly, however, it has a weakened sense, meaning merely "on the sides of". It may not be useless to point out that a "pore" was a passage, a tube (cf. τετμημένη in 29), and not merely a hole.

XXIX

κατὰ τὰς κοιλότητας τῶν ἀρτηριῶν καὶ τῶν
φλεβῶν παράκειται τροφὴ καὶ ἀνάδοσις
γίνεται αὐτῆς εἰς αὐτάς. * * καὶ μὴν κἀκεῖνο
35 δεῖ ὑπολαβεῖν, ὡς ἡ τροφὴ πᾶσα οὐ προστίθεται ἀναδιδομένη τῶι ὅλωι σώματι,
ἀλλὰ τὸ μὲν νόστιμον τὸ ἀπ᾽ αὐτῆς ἀναδίδοται καὶ προστίθεται τῶι σώματι, τὸ
δὲ ἀλλότριον καὶ σκυβαλῶδες χωριζό-
40 μενον εἰς ἔντερα διὰ τῶν ἀποπάτων ἀποκρίνεται. εἰ γάρ τοι πᾶσα ἡ λαμβανομένη τροφὴ
ἀναλαμβανομένη προσετίθετο, εἶτα
μηδεμία ἀπ᾽ αὐτῆς ἐγίνετο ἀπόκρισις, κἂν ἡμεῖς ὑπερφυεῖς κατά τε τὰ μεγέθη
45 καὶ τὰς ῥώμας ἐγινόμεθα, ἐπεὶ
ἀεὶ ἡμῖν προστίθεται· ἀλλ᾽ ἐπείπερ ἡ νόστιμος
[ἀεὶ τροφὴ τῆς] ἀλλοτρίας ἀποκρίνεται
........, μέτριοι κατὰ σώματά
ἐσμεν οὕτω. * τῶν δὲ ὑποδεδειγμένων
50 πρῶτόν ἐστιν τὸ περὶ τοῦ διὰ τῆς κύστεως
ἀποκρινομένου, περὶ οὗ ἰδία στάσις γεγένηται
καὶ παρὰ τοῖς ἀρχαίοις τῶν φιλοσόφων.
οἱ μὲν γὰρ εἶπον ἐν τῶι προσφερομένωι

XXX

ὑγρῶι ἐνυπάρχειν φύσιν διπλῆν τοιάν-
δε· καὶ νόστιμον καὶ φαῦλον ἐνεῖναι, ὧν τὸ μὲν
νόστιμον ἀναλαμβάνεσθαι διὰ τῶν ἀραιωμάτων καὶ προστίθεσθαι τοῖς σώμασιν, τὸ
5 δὲ φαῦλον φέρεσθαι εἰς τὸ κάτω καὶ διὰ
τὰς ἀπουρήσεις ἀποκρίνεσθαι εἰς τὸ ἐκτός.
οἱ δὲ ἔφασαν πᾶν μὲν ὑγρὸν ὁμοειδὲς αὐτὸ
ἑαυτῶι εἶναι, ἤδη δὲ κατὰ τὴν ἀνάληψιν
αὐτοῦ τὸ μὲν ἀναδιδόμενον προστίθεσθαι
10 τοῖς σώμασιν, τὸ δὲ μὴ ἀναδιδόμενον εἰς
τοὺς κατὰ τὴν κύστιν τόπους φέρεσθαι, ὅθεν διὰ
τῆς ἐν τούτοις ἐνυπαρχούσης δυνάμεως μεταβαλλόμενον
ἀποκρίνεται δριμύ τε καὶ ἁλμυρὸν γενόμενον.
ταύτηι γὰρ τὸ οὖρον ἑλκούσης δῆλον
15 ὅτι ἐστὶν δριμύ τε καὶ ἁλμυρόν. * πρὸς δὲ ἐκεῖ-

XXIX. 48.   D. would fill the gap with ὡς εἴρηται and add τὰ after κατά.
XXX. 14. ταύτη: D. says "hac via"; Cornford thought "by this δύναμις".

XXIX body, so that also along the hollows of the arteries and of the veins

nourishment is present and absorption of it takes place into them. * *

Further this too must be understood, that it is not all the food that is

added by absorption to the whole body; but the nourishing part from it

is absorbed and added to the body, while the unsuitable refuse separates

off into the intestines and is evacuated in the stools. For surely if

all food taken were absorbed and added to the body, and then no

evacuation from it took place, we too should become enormous in size

and strength, since additions to us are always taking place. But since

the nutritious food is always being separated from the unsuitable......

we have thus bodies of moderate size * but, of the things pointed out,

first is the section dealing with what is evacuated by way of the bladder,

XXX concerning which there has been a special controversy even among the

old scientists. For some have said that in the fluid taken a dual nature

exists of the following kind. Fluid they say contains both the beneficial

and the bad, of which the beneficial is absorbed through the pores and

is added to our bodies, while the bad is carried below and by urination

is excreted outside. Others have said that all fluid is homogeneous, and

only on its being taken is a part absorbed and added to our bodies,

while that which is not absorbed is carried to the parts about the region

of the bladder, whence, being changed by the power that is inherent

in these parts, it becomes pungent and salt and is excreted. For clearly

the urine is pungent and salt just because the bladder sucks it through

these parts. * With regard to that matter it must be said that it is to

XXX νο ῥητέον, ὅτι ἐπὶ τοῦ πρώτου ἐκκειμένου γίνονται οἱ πλείους τῶν ἀρχαίων.
καὶ εἰς τοῦτο ὑποδείγματι χρῶνται τῆι θαλάσσηι καὶ τῶι ἡλίωι· * οὗτος γὰρ τῶι ἄναμ-
20 μα νοερὸν ἐκ θαλάσσης εἶναι ἀπὸ
τοῦ νοστίμου τοῦ κατὰ τὴν θάλασσαν
τρέφεται, ἀναλαμβάνων μὲν τὸ λεπτόν, τὸ δὲ
ἀργότερον καὶ παχύτερον καὶ ἁλμυρὸν καταλεί-
πων ἐν τῆι θαλάσσηι. * ἀποφέρεται δὲ ὁμοίως
25 τοῦ προσφερομένου ὑγροῦ τὰ τρέφοντα ἡμᾶς·
ἀπὸ γὰρ τούτου τὸ μὲν νόστιμον καὶ λεπτὸν
ἀναδίδοται εἰς τὰ σώματα ἡμῶν, τὸ δὲ
φαυλότερον καὶ ἀργότερον σκὼρ γινόμενον διὰ
τὴν κύστιν εἰς τὸ ἐκτὸς ἀποκρίνεται.
30 τούτων οὕτως ἐκκειμένων ἀπορούμενοι μὲν
οὐκ ἔχομεν παγίως εἰπεῖν περὶ τοῦ ὑγροῦ
τοῦ ἀποκρινομένου κατὰ τὰ ἀπου[ρήματα], πότερον τὸ ἀλλότριόν ἐστιν τὸ ἀποκρινόμενον, ὃ ἐν-
υπῆρχεν τῶι ὑγρῶι καὶ ὃ φύσει δοκεῖ
35 ἐνυπάρχειν ἀχρεῖον ὑγρόν, ἢ ὃ γινόμενον ἐν τῆι
κύστει μεταβάλλεται πρὸς τὸ φαῦλον. * ἐ-
κεῖνο δὲ λέγομεν, ὅτι ἀπὸ τοῦ προσφερομένου
ὑγροῦ ἀποκρίνεται κατὰ τὰ σώματα
ὑγρὸν δριμύ τε καὶ ἁλμυρόν. * καὶ ταῦτα μὲν
40 περὶ τῆς διοικήσεως τῆς κατὰ τὴν κύστιν. * πει-
ρῶνται δὲ κατασκευάζειν, ὅτι ἀπὸ παντὸς τοῦ
σώματος συνεχεῖς γίνονται ἀποφοραί, λογιζόμενοι
ἀπό τινων τοιούτων· καὶ πρῶτον ἀπὸ τῶν ἀρωμάτων.
ἀρώματα γάρ, φασίν, εἰ πόρρω κέοιτο, ὀσφραινό-
45 μεθα τῶι σώματα φέρεσθαι ἀπ' αὐτῶν πρὸς ἡμᾶς.
τάχα δὲ πρὸς ταῦτ' ἐροῦσι ἀπὸ μὲν τῶν ἀρωμάτων
μὴ γίνεσθαι ἀποφορὰν σωμάτων, διατίθεσθαι
δὲ τὸν ἀέρα πρὸς τῶν ἀρωμάτων, τρόπον
δὲ τοῦτον κατὰ τὰς εἰσπνοὰς αἴσθησιν γίνεσθαι

---

18. Cf. Aetius, de placitis, II. 20, 16 (Doxogr. 351 b 9): Ἡράκλειτος καὶ
Ἑκαταῖος ἄναμμα νοερὸν τὸ ἐκ θαλάττης εἶναι τὸν ἥλιον. Ibidem, II.
20, 4 (349b 4) Κλεάνθης ἄναμμα νοερὸν τὸ ἐκ θαλάττης τὸν ἥλιον. Arius
Didymus, fr. 34 apud Stob. Ecl. eth. I. 26 (Doxogr. 467, 17): Χρύσιππος τὸ
ἀθροισθὲν ἔξαμμα μετὰ τὸν ἥλιον νοερὸν ἐκ τοῦ ἀπὸ τῶν ποτίμων ὑδάτων
ἀναθυμιάματος· διὸ καὶ τούτοις τρέφεσθαι.

XXX the first opinion here indicated that the majority of the ancients incline. As an analogous case bearing upon the point they make use of the sea and the sun. * For the sun, by reason of its being an intelligent ball of fire out of the sea, is nourished from the nutritious part in the sea, taking in the part that is fine, but leaving in the sea the more sluggish, the grosser and the salt portion. * In a similar manner from the fluid that we take in there is taken away the parts that nourish us. For from this fluid the nutritive and fine part is absorbed into our bodies, while the inferior and more sluggish becomes refuse and is eliminated outside through the bladder. With this exposition of the matter, we are still at a loss and cannot say for certain about the fluid that is eliminated as urine, whether the eliminated part is the unsuitable part, which was originally present in the fluid and is thought to be present as a naturally useless fluid; or whether it is that which, when it gets into the bladder, changes for the worse. * But this we do say, that from the fluid taken in there is excreted from our bodies a fluid that is pungent and salt. * So much for the physiology of the bladder. *

29   But they try to prove that from all the body continuous emanations take place, drawing conclusions from certain observations such as the following. Firstly from spices. For spices, they say, should they be placed at a distance, we smell because bodies are carried from them to us. But perhaps they will urge in reply that there does not take place an emanation of bodies from the spices, but that the air is put into a certain condition by the spices, and in this way as we inhale we become

19, 20.   ἄναμμα is a red-hot mass.
40 and 46.   What is the subject? B. and S. have "man".
47, 50.   For μὴ where classical Greek would have οὐ see p. 33.

XXX 50 ἡμῖν τῶν ἀπὸ τῶν ἀρωμάτων διαπνοῶν καὶ μὴ
εἶναι ἀποφοράν. * * νωθρὸν δὲ λίαν φαίνεται
τοῦτο· σώματα γάρ ἐστιν κατὰ τὸ λόγωι θεωρητὸν

XXXI τὰ ἀποσπώμενα ἀπὸ τῶν ἀρωμάτων. καὶ τοῦτο
δῆλον ἐπὶ τῶν πεπαλαιωμένων ἀραιωμάτων·
ταῦτα γὰρ ἀσθενῆ καὶ οὐκ ἐνεργοῦσαν ἴσχει
τὴν δύναμιν διὰ τὸ πολλὴν γεγενῆσθαι ἀπ' αὐ-
5   τῶν διὰ τὸν χρόνον ἀποφοράν, ἐξ ὧν συνάγεται
τὸ λεγόμενον. * * καὶ ἀπὸ τῶν κρεῶν δὲ τἀτὸ ὑπομιμνήσκουσι λέγοντες τὰ μὲν ἕωλα κουφότερα εἶναι
καὶ ὀλιγοτροφώτερα, τὰ δὲ πρόσφατα βαρύτερα
καὶ πολυτροφώτερα. καὶ τοῦτο δῆλον ἐπὶ τῆς
10   αὐτοψίας· σταθὲν γὰρ τὸ ἕωλον κρέας κατα-
λήψηι κουφότερον, τὸ δὲ πρόσφατον βαρύτερον.
τίνος αἰτίας γινομένης; δῆλον ὅτι τῶι ἀπὸ μὲν τῶν ἑώλων
πολλὴν γεγονέναι ἀποφοράν, ἀπὸ δὲ τῶν προσφάτων
ὀλίγον, καὶ μὴ διαφέρειν ἢ κατὰ τὸ αἰσθητὸν
15   ἀπὸ τοῦ ὑποκειμένου ποιεῖσθαι ἀφαίρεσιν ἢ κατὰ
τὸ λόγωι θεωρητόν. * * καὶ μὴν καὶ ἀπὸ τῶν ἄρτων
τἀτὸ κατασκευάζουσιν· οἱ γὰρ θερμότεροι βαρύτεροί
τε καὶ πολυτροφώτεροι, οἱ δὲ ψυχρότεροι
κουφότεροι καὶ ὀλιγοτροφώτεροι διὰ τὴν αὐτὴν
20   αἰτίαν. καὶ ταὐτὰ πιστοῦσιν οἱ ἀλεῖπται· οὐκ ἄν
ποτε γὰρ προσέφερον τοῖς ἀθληταῖς θερμούς τε
ἄρτους καὶ πρόσφατα κρέα, εἰ μὴ βαρύτερα ἦν
καὶ πολυτροφώτερα, τοὺς δὲ ψυχροτέρους
ἄρτους καὶ τὰ ἕωλα τῶν κρεῶν ἐξέκλεινον,
25   εἰ μὴ ὀλιγότροφα καὶ κοῦφα ὑπῆρχεν. * * πρὸς τούτους τοὺς
λόγους ἀντιφέρονται οἱ Ἐμπειρικοὶ λέγοντες· ''οὐκ εἴ
τι ἀπό τινος ἀφαιρεῖται, ἐκεῖνο ὀφείλει κοῦφον γίνεσθαι, οὐδ' εἴ τί τινι προστίθεται, ἐκεῖνο βαρύτερον γίνεται, ἀλλ' ἔστιν ὅτε προσθέσεως γινομένης τὸ
30   ὑποκείμενον κατασκευάζεται κουφότερον, ἔστιν δ' ὅτε
καὶ ἀφαιρέσεως γενομένης τὸ ὑποκείμενον
γίνεται βαρύτερον ὡς ἐπὶ τῶν ἀσκῶν καὶ ἐπὶ τῶν

XXXI. 2.   ἀραιωμάτων is clearly a slip for ἀρωμάτων.
14.   Perhaps ὀλίγην.
29.   Perhaps γενομένης.

XXX conscious of the breaths from the spices, and there is no emanation. * * But this explanation is manifestly very stupid, for the tiny fragments from the spices are bodies falling under the perceptive power of the reason. XXXI This becomes plain if we take the case of stale spices. For these are faint and have lost their active properties because in course of time the emanation from them has grown considerable, facts from which their statement is deduced (?) * * They make the same observation about meat, saying that high meat is lighter and less nourishing, while fresh is heavier and more nourishing. This becomes clear on personal inspection. For high meat on being weighed you will find to be lighter and fresh meat heavier. What is the reason? Surely it is because from the high meat the emanation has been great, but from the fresh slight, and because it makes no difference whether a perceptible removal from the object takes place or whether it is one that can only be inferred by reason. * * Moreover they make the same inferences from loaves of bread. The warmer are heavier and more nourishing, the cooler lighter and less nourishing for the same reason. Confirmatory evidence comes from the gymnastic trainers. For they would never give to athletes warm loaves and fresh meat, were they not heavier and more nourishing, nor would they avoid cooler loaves and high meat were not these of little nutritive value and light by nature. * * These arguments are opposed by the Empirics, who say that "becoming light does not depend upon a part being taken from a thing, nor does the addition of one thing to another necessarily make the latter heavier. Sometimes on the addition of something the object is made lighter, and sometimes too on the subtraction of a part the object becomes heavier, as in the

XXX. 51. κατὰ τὸ λόγῳ θεωρητόν, a common phrase in this part of *Anonymus*, might be rendered "by the light of reason", or "with the mind's eye". Perhaps the most idiomatic equivalent would be simply "invisible", or "inferred". I have varied my translation to suit the context.
XXXI. 17. What is the subject? B. and S. translate "wiesen sie".
26. The Empirics: see for these Clifford Allbutt, *Greek Medicine at Rome*, pp. 166–170.

XXXI τετελευτηκότων ζώιων καὶ ἀνθέων." * * καὶ ᾱ
μὲν τοῦ ἀσκοῦ ὑπομιμνήσκουσιν· "ὁ ἀσκὸς
35 γενόμενος χωρὶς πνεύματος βαρύτερός ἐστιν, πληρωθεὶς
δὲ πνεύματος κουφότερος γίνεται. καὶ τὰ ζῶια
ἐκ β̄ τούτων συνέστηκεν, ψυχῆς τε καὶ σώματος,
καὶ ὅτε μὲν ἀμφότερα ταῦτα πάρεστιν, κουφότερόν ἐστιν
τὸ ζῶιον, ὅτε δὲ ἀφανίζεται ἀπὸ τοῦ σώματος
40 ἡ ψυχή, βαρύτερον γίνεται τὸ σῶμα." * "καὶ μήν, φασίν,
ὅτι ἔστιν σῶμα ἡ ψυχή, οἱ πλείους τῶν φιλοσόφων
λέγουσι. καὶ ἀσώματον δὲ αὐτὴν ἀπολεί-
42a ποντες οὐσίαν ἤ τινα αὐτὴν ἔχειν ἔφασαν, ὡς ἡ θυρὶς ἀφαιρέσει
μείζων γίνεται, προσθέσει δὲ μικροτέρα.
φανερὸν οὖν τοιγάρτοι ἐκ τούτων, ὡς κατὰ ἀφαίρεσιν
45 γίνεται βαρύτης καὶ κατὰ πρόσθεσιν κουφότης, ὡς ὑπε-
δείξαμεν." * * λείαν δ᾽ ἐστὶν οὗτος ὁ λόγος μωρός τε
καὶ ἀπατητικός, ὡς ἀποδείξομεν. ᾱ μὲν ἀποδείξομεν οὕτως· τινὸς γὰρ ἀφαιρέσει λέγομέν τινι
πρόσθεσιν γίνεσθαι, ἀλλὰ οὐχὶ τούτου τῆς προσθέσεως
50 ὁ αὐτὸς λόγος· προστίθεμεν γὰρ τῆι θυρίδι,
ἀφαιροῦμεν δὲ τοῦ τοίχου. * * εἶτα καὶ ἐπὶ τῆς
ψυχῆς διὰ βραχέων λέγομεν, ὡς ἡ ψυχὴ αἰτία ἐστὶν
γινομένη τῆς κουφότητος καὶ ..τικνιασε ....
.... τῆς κουφότητος· * * δι᾽ ἣν αἰτίαν παρού-

XXXII σης μὲν τῆς ψυχῆς κοῦφόν ἐστιν τὸ ζῶιον, ὅτι καὶ πνεῦμα
ἡ ψυχή, τὸ δὲ πνεῦμα κοῦφον τὴν φύσιν
†τοπνευμα†. πνευματικὴ δὲ καὶ ἡ ψυχή· τοιαύ-
τη δὲ ὑπάρχουσα εὐλόγως παροῦσα μὲν κοῦφον παρέχει τὸ ζῶιον,
5 ἀποῦσα δὲ βαρύτερον· * οὕτως γὰρ ὑπὸ τῆς ψυχῆς
βαστάζεται τὸ ὅλον σῶμα. γίνεται δέ... λεγειν τοῦτο μὲν
†αποτωναλων† ἀπὸ τῶν ἄλλων δυνάμεων, αὗται δὲ ἀπὸ τῶν κεινήσεων. * κεινεῖται γὰρ τὸ ὅλον σῶμα τῆς

XXXI. 33.   Simplicius ad Ar. de caelo, 313 b 44 K.: τὸ δὲ τὸν ἀέρα ἐν τῇ
ὁλότητι τῇ ἑαυτοῦ μὴ ἔχειν βάρος καὶ ὁ Πτολεμαῖος ἐκ τοῦ αὐτοῦ τεκμη-
ρίου τοῦ κατὰ τὸν ἀσκὸν δείκνυσιν οὐ μόνον πρὸς τὸ βαρύτερον εἶναι τὸν
πεφυσημένον ἀσκὸν τοῦ ἀφυσήτου, ὅπερ ἐδόκει Ἀριστοτέλει, ἀντιλέγων,
ἀλλὰ καὶ κουφότερον αὐτὸν γενέσθαι φυσηθέντα βουλόμενος. ἐγὼ δὲ
πειραθεὶς μετὰ τῆς δυνατῆς ἀκριβείας τὸν αὐτὸν εὗρον σταθμὸν ἀφυσήτου
τε ὄντος καὶ φυσηθέντος τοῦ ἀσκοῦ.

42a.   ἥντινα ("whatever it is") Hackforth.
49.   Cornford would put a full stop at τούτου.

XXXI case of bladders and of dead animals and flowers." * * And the first evidence they cite is that of a bladder. "A bladder emptied of air is heavier, and filled with air it becomes lighter. Animals too are composed of these two things, soul and body. When both these components are present, the animal is lighter; when the soul disappears from the body, the body becomes heavier." * "Furthermore," they say, "the majority of scientists assert that the soul is body. And even when making out that soul is bodiless they have declared that it has some sort of essence, as the window becomes greater when bricks are taken away, and smaller when they are added. Accordingly therefore it is shown by this evidence that weight comes on subtraction and lightness on addition, as we have indicated." * * This reasoning, however, is very stupid and misleading, as we shall show. Our first point will be that by taking away a part of a thing we say that something is added to another thing, but the same argument does not apply to the addition of this thing. For when we add to the window, we take away from the wall. * * Then too in the case of the soul we briefly put it that the soul by its presence is cause of the lightness....................

......Through which cause when the soul is present the animal is XXXII light, because the soul is also air, and air is light by nature. The soul also is of an air-like nature. Such being the soul's nature, it is reasonable that its presence makes the animal light, while its absence makes the animal heavier. * For in this way the whole body is supported by the soul. The body comes into being as the result of the other powers, while they are the result of movements. * For the whole

XXXI. 42a. The ἦ seems pointless. D. suggests δυ (=δύναμιν): "that soul has some power". Perhaps δή: "has *some* sort of essence".

49, 50. Obscurely put. Perhaps the argument is that adding to the window makes smaller, not the window but the wall, while adding soul to the body makes (not something else but) the body lighter. Cornford's punctuation would give: "It is a subtraction from *A*, not from *B*, that adds to *B*. Similarly with addition."

XXXII. 3. πνευματική κ.τ.λ. This is perhaps a lecturer's repetition; it is certainly unnecessary.

7, 8. Probably κείνης ("of the soul") has fallen out between κεινήσεων and κεινεῖται. But the sentence is very obscure.

XXXII

ψυχῆς διὰ τοῦ γεώδους καὶ ἀερώδους καὶ
10 διαβασταζούσης αὐτά· οὕτως ἐκεῖνο τείνεται
ἄνω· γινομένης γὰρ αὐτῆς τῆς ψυχῆς γίνεται·
διὸ δὴ καὶ ῥητέον, ὅτι οὐχ ὅταν τινὸς γένηται πρόσθεσις, ἐκεῖνο γίνεται βαρύτερον, ἀλλὰ ἐὰν βαρέος τινός
τινι γένηται πρόσθεσις, ἐκεῖνο γίνεται βαρύτερον.
15 ἡ δὲ ψυχὴ τοσοῦτον ἀπέχει τοῦ εἶναι βαρεῖα,
ὥστε καὶ τὸ φύσει καταρρέπον κουφίζειν καὶ
βαστάζειν. ταύτης οὖν παρούσης δεόντως κοῦφόν ἐστιν τὸ ζῶιον. ὅταν μέντοι γε
ἀφανισθῆι ἡ ψυχή, τῶι μηκέτι παρεῖναι
20 τὸ κουφίζον μηδὲ αἰωροῦν λοιπὸν βαρέ†ι†α
φαίνεται εὐλόγως τὰ νεκρὰ ταύτης αἰτίαι.
καὶ ἐπὶ τῶν ἀσκῶν δὲ πεπληρωμένων τοῦ πνεύματος κουφότης
καταλαμβάνεται τῶι τοῦτο κοῦφον ὂν κου-
φίζειν τὸν ἀσκόν. ὅταν δὲ μὴ παρῆι τὸ πνεῦμα,
25 βαρὺς γίνεται ὁ ἀσκὸς τῶι ἐστερῆσθαι τοῦ κου-
φίζοντος αἰτίου. * ἀλλὰ γὰρ διὰ ταὐτὸ γίνεται καὶ τὰ τῶν
θερμῶν ἄρτων· καὶ ψυχρότεροι μὲν κουφότεροι, θερμότεροι δὲ
βαρύτεροί εἰσιν· καὶ βαρύτεροι μὲν οὗτοι τῶι μηδέ-
πω πολλὴν ἀποφορὰν γεγενῆσθαι ἀπ' αὐτῶν,
30 οἱ δὲ ψυχροὶ κοῦφοί εἰσιν τῶι ὅλης τῆς ὕλης
ἱκανὴν ἀποφορὰν γεγενῆσθαι. * ἔτι δὲ καὶ
ἀπὸ τούτων διδάσκουσιν, ὡς γίνονται ὄντως ἀποφοραὶ κατὰ τὸ λόγωι θεωρητὸν καὶ α... αἰτίων ὑπαρχόντων·
τὰ γὰρ ὑγρὰ τὰ ἐν ἀγγείοις τισὶν ὑπομείναν-
35 τα ποσοὺς χρόνους ἐλάττω καταισθάνεται.
καὶ ἀπὸ τῶν χυλῶν τἀτὸ γίνεται· ἐνίοτε γὰρ ὑπὸ ἡλίου
ἢ ἄλλων τινῶν συνξηρανθέντες ἐπί τινος
φαίνονται. τίνος γινομένου; τῶι δηλονότι λεπτὴν ἀποφορὰν γεγενῆσθαι ἀπ' αὐτῶν τοῦ λεπτομερεστέρου,
40 ὑπομονὴν δὲ τοῦ γεωδεστέρου, ἃ δὴ αὐτὰ γίνεται
καὶ ἐπὶ τῶν ἀναπλασσομένων κολλυρίων. * καὶ
ἐπὶ τὰ φυτὰ δὲ μεταβαίνουσιν καὶ λέγουσιν

---

9. ἀερώδους or πυρώδους may be the true reading. A line seems to have
fallen out after καί. 20. For αἰωροῦν D suggests αἰωρεῖν.
"30 et 33. extrema dubia, αἰτίων explicat V 36 sqq." (D.).
33. Before αἰτίων read ἄνευ.
35. καταισθάνεται (passive) is dubious, but all the letters except θ are
clear.

XXXII body is moved because the soul, through the earthy element and the airy element, supports them. So the body reaches upwards, for its coming into being depends upon the coming into being of the soul itself. For this reason then it must also be said that it is not an addition to a body that makes it heavier, but the addition of a heavy thing that makes it heavier. But the soul is so far from being heavy that it actually lightens and supports that which naturally tends to sink. When therefore soul is present the animal of necessity is light. When, however, the soul has disappeared, because there is no longer present that which lightens and lifts, hereafter the dead bodies appear heavy with good reason because of the soul. And in the case of the bladders which have been filled with air, lightness is found because air, being light, lightens the bladder. But when the air is no longer present, the bladder becomes heavy because it has been deprived of the cause that lightens it. * But in truth it is for the same reason that warm loaves get their peculiar properties, and are lighter when cooler and heavier when warmer. The latter are heavier because no great emanation has as yet taken place from them, while the cold are light because considerable emanation has taken place from the whole of their substance. * Furthermore the following facts lead them to maintain that emanations, appealing to the perception of the reason, really do take place without pre-existing cause. For liquids that have been left for some time in certain vessels are perceived to be less in volume. The same emanation takes place from juices. For at times they plainly dry up upon a thing when exposed to the sun or to similar influences. What takes place? It is clear that it is because a fine emanation of the finer component has taken place from the juices, while the more earthy part has remained behind, which is the very thing that takes place when poultices are plastered on. * Then they turn their attention to plants, saying that when freshly cut

9. Perhaps "fiery" (πυρώδους). The sentence is hard to understand. Does it mean that soul, pervading the bodily elements, rears these into a structure? "For soul is form and doth the body make." If so, perhaps for αὐτά we should read αὐτό, in spite of ἐκεῖνο. See also B. and S., p. 49.

37. ἐπί τινος: perhaps "to a certain extent". The subjects of the verbs in this part of the argument cannot be determined with certainty [διδάσκουσι (32), μεταβαίνουσι (42), πιστοῦσι (48), λέγουσι (49) and συλλέγουσι (55)]. But it is probably the followers or the opponents of Erasistratus. But does the lecturer (writer) agree with the theory of pores and emanations? It would be of great interest to know. See pp. 7, 8.

XXXII

τὰ μὲν παραυτὰ ἀποτμηθέντα βαρύτερα εἶναι,
τὰ δὲ ποσοὺς ὑπομείναντα χρόνους κουφότερα
45   ὡς ἐπὶ τῆς θριδακείης, ἐπὶ τῶν ἀνθέων·
ταῦτα γὰρ πάντα διὰ τὴν ἀποφορὰν ῥυσόκαρφα
κατασκευάζεται. ἐγ δὴ τούτων καὶ τῶν τούτοις
παραπλησίων πιστοῦσιν, ὡς ἀποφορὰ γίνεται ἀπὸ τοῦ
σώματος. * * πρὸς τοῦτον τὸν λόγον λέγουσιν·
50   εἰ ἡ ἀποφορὰ αἰτία ἐστὶν τῆς ῥυσότητος, ἐχρῆν μὴ
μόνον κατὰ τὴν ἀπότμηξιν ῥυσοῦσθαι
τὰ προκείμενα, ἀλλά τι καὶ ἐπὶ τῶν δενδρῶν·
καὶ γὰρ καὶ ἀπὸ τοῦ δένδρους ἀπουσία γίνεται·
οὐ γίνεται δὲ τοῦτο· οὐκ ἄρα ἡ ἀποφορὰ αἰτία ἐστὶ
55   τῆς ῥυσότητος. * * συλλέγουσι δὲ οὗτοι

XXXIII

τὸ ἀνὰ λόγον· γίνεται μὲν γὰρ καὶ ἐπὶ τῶν δενδρῶν ἀποφορὰ τῶν ἀνθέων †ου† πλείων, †αλλα δενδρων† ἐπὶ
δὲ τῶν ἀφειρημένων οὐ πλείων. * καὶ ἐπὶ μὲν †των επι† τῶι
δένδρει καὶ ἡ κείνησις αὐτὴ ἀναλοῖ πλείω καὶ
5   ἔτι ἡ θερμασία ἀναλοῖ ἱκανά, * ἐπὶ δὲ τῶν ἀποτετμη-
μένων καὶ μὴ ὑπὸ φύσεως διοικουμένων ἐλάσσω
τῶι μήτε κείνησιν μήτε θερμότητά τινα εἶναι ἐπ᾽ αὐτῶν.
τίς οὖν ἡ αἰτία, παρ᾽ ἣν τὰ μὲν ἀποτμηθέντα ξηραίνεται, τὰ δὲ ἐπὶ τῶι δένδρει οὐ ξηραίνεται; * σα-
10   φὴς δὲ αὕτη καὶ φαινομένη· τὰ μὲν γὰρ ἐπὶ τῶι δένδρει οὐ ξηραίνεται τῶι πρὸς λόγον τῆς ἀποφορᾶς
γίνεσθαι καὶ τὴν πρόσθεσιν. * * τὰ δὲ ἀποτμηθέντα ξηραίνεται τῶι μηκέτι γίνεσθαι ὡς αὐτὰ πρόσθεσιν, ἐξ ὧν σαφὲς
ὡς καὶ ἀπὸ τῶν φυτῶν γίνεται ἀποφορά. * καὶ ἐπὶ τὰ
15   ἄλογα δὲ τῶν ζώιων καταβαίνουσι. λαμβάνουσιν γὰρ τοὺς
θηρευ-
τὰς κύνας, ὡς οὗτοι τῆι ῥινηλασίαι συνθη-
ρεύουσι τὰ θηρία τρόπωι τούτωι· παραγίνον-
ται ἐπὶ τὰς ἀτραπούς, δι᾽ ὧν κεχώρηκεν
τὰ θηρία, καὶ τῶν ἀτραπῶν ὀδμωμένων
20   χωροῦσιν ἐπὶ τὴν θήραν. τίνος αἰτίας γινομένης; δῆλον ὅτι τῆς ἀπὸ τῶν θηρίων ἀποφορᾶς προσκαθιζούσης πρὸς τὰς ἀτραπούς. ταύτηι δὴ
καὶ ἐν τοῖς καταξήροις τόποις θῆραι οὐ γίνονται,

XXXIII. 13. ὡσαυτά M. Fränkel.

XXXII they are heavier, but when they have been left for a while they are lighter, as in the case of lettuce and of flowers. For these in all cases shrivel up because of the emanation. By this and similar evidence they support their contention that emanation takes place from the body. * * To this argument they reply. If the emanation is the cause of the shrivelling, the objects under discussion ought to have shrivelled not only when cut off, but also to a certain extent when growing on trees; for in truth a tree too loses its substance. But this does not happen. Therefore the cause of shrivelling cannot XXXIII be the emanation. * * Their opponents appeal to proportion. For even on the trees there takes place a considerable emanation from their flowers, but an inconsiderable one from flowers that have been cut off. * And on the tree the mere motion gets rid of a considerable number and heat too gets rid of more than a few; * but in the case of those cut off and no longer maintained by nature there are fewer losses, because there is neither motion nor any heat to affect them. What then is the cause why the flowers cut off wither, while those on the tree do not? * This is plain and manifest. The flowers on the tree do not wither because the addition that takes place is in proportion to the emanation. * * But those that have been cut off wither, because an addition no longer reaches them. From which facts it is clear that from plants also emanation takes place. * They pass on also to the irrational animals. For they instance hounds, which in tracking by scent help in hunting wild beasts in the following way. They make their way to the tracks along which the beasts have passed, and smell the tracks while pursuing their quarry. What is the cause of this? Clearly because the emanation from the beasts settles on the tracks. This of course is the very reason why there is no hunting in parched

XXXII. 50 ff.   The argument is: If emanations take place from both cut-off flowers and flowers still on the plant, and if emanations cause shrivelling, why do not flowers shrivel when on the plant but only when cut off?

XXXIII. 2.   Is τῶν ἀνθέων subjective or objective genitive, "emanations from their flowers" or "shedding of their flowers"?

XXXIII   ἐν μέντοι γε τοῖς χαυνοτέροις. καὶ ἡ αἰτία πρό-
25   κειται, ἐπειδήπερ τὰ ἀπὸ τῶν θηρίων σώματα
  ἀποσκιδνάμενα προσπείπτοντα μὲν γῆι ἀπο-
  κρότωι καὶ †μῆ† καταξήρωι †τη† κατασκίδναται,
  χαυνοτέραι δὲ προσπεσόντα καὶ παραδεχομένηι
  φυλάσσεται καὶ διαμένει. ταύτηι δὴ οἱ θηρευ-
30   ταὶ κύνες χωροῦντες καὶ ὀσφρώμενοι τῆς
  ἀποφορᾶς τῆς ἀπὸ τῶν θηρίων τῶι περισώζεσθαι
  αὐτήν, εἶτα χωρήσαντες καταλαμβάνου-
  σι τὸ θηρίον καὶ αἱροῦσι. * ταύτηι δὴ καὶ ἐπὶ τῶν
  ὑετῶν οὐ γίνονται ῥινηλασίαι κατὰ λόγον· ἐξαφανίζων γὰρ ὁ
  ὄμβρος
35   τὰ ἀπὸ τῶν θηρίων σκιδνάμενα σώματα κω-
  λυτήριος γίνεται τῆς θήρας. καὶ τούτωι μὲν τῶι
  τρόπωι γίνονται αἱ θῆραι. * * μάλιστα δὲ γίνονται καὶ ἐὰν
  σκύλακες
  †κες† ἕπωνται τοῖς θηρίοις καὶ ἐὰν νέα ἦι· ἀπα-
  λώτερα γὰρ ὄντα πλείονα τὴν ἀποφορὰν ποιεῖ·
40   οὕτως γε ἡ γῆ πλείονα δεχομένη τὴν
  ἀποφορὰν ῥαιδίως σημαίνει τοῖς κυσὶ τὰ θηρία.
  εἰ δὲ ταῦτα, φανερὸν ὡς γίνονταί τινες
  ἀποφοραὶ καὶ ἀπὸ τῶν ἀλόγων ζώιων. * * πρὸς δὲ τούτοις
  καὶ Ἐρασίστρατος πειρᾶται κατασκευάζειν τὸ προτεθέν.
45   εἰ γὰρ λάβοι τις ζῶιον οἷον ὄρνιθα ἤ τι τῶν παραπλησίων, καταθοῖτο δὲ τοῦτο ἐν λέβητι
  ἐπί τινας χρόνους μὴ δοὺς τροφήν, ἔπειτα
  σταθμήσαιτο σὺν τοῖς σκυβάλοις τοῖς αἰσθητῶς
  κεκενωμένοις, εὑρήσει παρὰ πολὺ ἔλασ-
50   σον τοῦτο τῶι σταθμῶι τῶι δηλονότι πολλὴν ἀποφορὰν γεγενῆσθαι κατὰ τὸ λόγωι θεωρητόν. * *
  ἀλλὰ γὰρ καὶ ἐπὶ τὸν ἄνθρωπον μεταβαίνοντες
  ποιοῦνται τὸν λόγον· οἵ τε γὰρ πιόντες ἀρώματα
  καὶ οἱ σκορδοφαγήσαντες ὅμοιον ἔχουσι
55   τὸ διὰ τῶν ἱδρώτων κενούμενον τοῖς προσενη-

XXXIV   νεγμένοις, ὡς ἂν δὴ ἀποφορᾶς γεγενημένης
  κατὰ τὸ λόγωι θεωρητὸν ἀπὸ τῶν προσενηνεγμένων·
  εἰ δὲ ταῦτα ἐν τῆι ἡμετέραι συγκρίσει ὄντα
  ἀποφέρεται κατὰ τὸ λόγωι θεωρητὸν καὶ κατὰ τὸ αἰσθητόν,
5   καὶ ἐκτὸς ὄντα ἡμῶν ἕξει σώματά τινα ἀπορ-

XXXIII regions, but only over loose soil. The reason is ready to hand; for the particles that are dispersed from the wild beasts, when they fall on land that is hard and very dry, are dissipated, but once they have fallen on loose, receptive land they are preserved, and so persist. In this way then hounds go on smelling the emanation from the wild beasts because it is being preserved, and then after tracking it down they come upon the beast and capture it. * Wherefore too it is only natural in times of rain there is no tracking by scent. For the shower, washing away the particles that are scattered from the wild beasts, puts a stop to the chase. In this manner, then, hunting is carried on. * * They succeed most if the hounds that follow be puppies and the hunted beasts be young. For the young, being softer, send off a more copious emanation, and so the ground, receiving a more copious emanation, easily directs the hounds to the wild beasts. If this be so, clearly irrational animals also give off certain emanations. * *

30   In addition to all this Erasistratus too attempts to establish the point thus. If one were to take a creature, such as a bird or something of the sort, and were to place it in a pot for some time without giving it any food, and then were to weigh it with the excrement that visibly has been passed, he will find that there has been a great loss of weight, plainly because, perceptible only to the reason, a copious emanation has taken place. * * But turning their attention to man also, they proceed thus in their argument. Those who have drunk spices, and those who have eaten garlic, give evacuations through sweats

XXXIV that are like what they have taken, a fact implying that an emanation has taken place, perceptible to reason, from the things taken. But if these things in our system are given off so as to be perceptible both by reason and by the senses, bodies outside us too will give off some

XXXIV

ρέοντα ἀπ' αὐτῶν. * * ὁ δὲ Ἀσκληπιάδης πειρᾶται
κατὰ τὸν τόπον καινολογεῖν· τὰ γὰρ ἀρώματά φησιν
καὶ τὰ σκόροδα τὴν ἰδίαν ποιότητα ἀποβάλλειν
ἐν τῆι ἡμετέραι συνκρίσει γενόμενα. εἰ γὰρ συνέσω-
10   ζεν ἐν ταῖς ἡμετέραις συγκρίσεσι τὰς ποιότητας,
ἐνῆν καὶ ἡμᾶς καὶ αἰσθάνεσθαι καὶ συναντιλαμβάνεσθαι
.........υ γὰρ ἐπὶ λελυμένης καθ' ὅλον
.... τὰ ληφθέντα καὶ ἐξαιματω-
θέντα........θεν μόριον τοῦ σώματος
15   ....ρας εἰ τοῦτο
.... καὶ τοῖς μυκτῆρσι
..... γίνεται ανεν...... ἡμῶν, ἐπειδήπερ
...... ἡ ποιότης ἐν τοῖς ἡμετέροις σώμασίν ἐστιν
.... αἰσθανόμεθα γὰρ
20   .... ὅτι δὲ αἱ ποιότητες............. τῶι σώματι δὲ γενηθ.....
.........ἀποφερομένας αἰτι... ὑπο
...............ει * ἴσως δέ τις ἐρεῖ
... συνδια.......ες τῶν λαμβανομένων
25   ....τῆς ποιότητος
.... τῆς ἐν τοῖς σώμασιν
ο........μέναις φλεψὶν ἀναλύεται καὶ ἀπόλ-
λυται........... ἐπὶ φανερὰ γένη
.οι τα.λ.ι σωμ....ται καὶ περισώζεται
30   ..λα. * * πρὸς μέντοι τοῦτον πειρῶνταί τινες
ἀντιλέγειν, φέρεσθαι μὲν καὶ ἐπὶ τοὺς μυκτῆρας τὸ ἀναθυμιατὸν καὶ ἐπὶ τὰ λοιπὰ μέρη
τοῦ σώματος, μηδὲν δὲ ἐπὶ πλεῖον κακοῦν
τὴν αἴσθησιν καὶ κωλυτήριον γίνεσθαι τῆς
35   ἀντιλήψεως τῶν ἐδεσθέντων. * * ὃν τρόπον
καὶ οἱ βυρσοδέψαι· οὗτοι γὰρ κεκακωμένην ἴσχοντες τὴν αἴσθησιν οὐδὲν παραποδίζονται
κατὰ τὴν ὀδμήν· * τὸν αὐτὸν καὶ ἀπὸ τῶν ἐδεσ-
τῶν κακουμένη αἴσθησις †ουκαντιλαμβ†
40   οὐκ ἀντιλαμβάνεται τῆς δυνάμεως τῆς ἀπ' αὐτῶν.
οὐ πιθανῶς δὲ οὐδ' οὗτοι ἐπιχειροῦσιν †προς αυτον†·
ἡμεῖς δέ φαμεν πρὸς τὸν Ἀσκληπιάδη, διότι ἡ αἴσθησις τῶν ἐν ἡμῖν οὐκ ἀντιλαμβάνεται διὰ τὸ μὴ

---

29. Perhaps σωματοῦται.

XXXIV particles from them. * * But Asclepiades attempts a novel theory about the place. For he asserts that spices and garlic lose their peculiar properties when they have been taken into our system. For if they had preserved their qualities in our systems, it would have been possible for us too both to perceive them and to apprehend their nature....

.... since the quality is in our bodies.

31 However, in reply to him certain thinkers attempt to assert that the scent is carried both to the nostrils and to the other parts of the body, but while doing no further harm to sensation yet hinders the apprehension of the things eaten * * as is the case also with tanners. For they, though having their sense vitiated, yet retain unimpaired the power of smell. * Similarly too a sense that is being vitiated by the foods taken does not feel the strong quality they give off. But this attempted explanation too possesses no plausibility.

32 Our own reply to Asclepiades is that the sense does not apprehend

33. μηδέν: see p. 33.
35. "Post τρόπον non extitit ἔχουσιν, at audiendum, utique ὃν τρόπον... ὀδμὴν per anacoluthian est pro protasi, cuius apodosis sequitur v. 38 sqq." D. The point being argued seems to be: Why do we not smell strong-smelling foods once they are eaten? (a) Is the property lost in our bodies? (b) Is the power of smelling lost owing to the overpowering nature of the smell? (c) Is the smell removed from the cognizance of the sense-organ?
38. It is assumed that τρόπον has been lost before τὸν αὐτόν.

XXXIV ὑποπείπτειν αὐτῆι αὐτά. ὃν γὰρ τρόπον τὸ πεσσό-
45 μενον ἐν οἰκείωι τόπωι δεῖ εἶναι, ἵνα πέψηι,
καὶ ὃν τρόπον τὸ ἐξαιματούμενον δεῖ ἐν οἰκείωι
τόπωι γενέσθαι εἰς τὸ ἐξαιματωθῆναι, οὕτω καὶ
τὸ ὁδμώμενον ἐν οἰκείωι τόπωι δεῖ εἶναι
εἰς τὸ ὀσφρηθῆναι. τὰ δὲ ἐν ἡμῖν ὑπάρχοντα μὴ ὑπο-
50 πείπτοντα τῆι αἰσθήσει εἰκότως ἐγλανθάνει
αὐτήν· δι᾽ ἣν αἰτίαν τῶν εὐωδῶν λαμβανομένων
ἡ αἴσθησις οὐ καταλαμβάνει τὰς τούτων ποιότητας.
καὶ πρὸς μὲν τὸν Ἀσκληπιάδη ταῦτα. * * λέγουσι

XXXV δὲ καὶ ἀποφέρεσθαι ἀπὸ τῶν ἡμετέρων σωμάτων
θερμότητα καὶ ὑγρότητα. καὶ ὡς ἡ μὲν θερμότης
ἀποφέρεται, ὑπομιμνήσκουσι διὰ τούτων· τὰ
ἱμάτια ψυχρότερα περιβαλόμενοι θερμότερα
εὑρίσκομεν, ὡς ἂν δὴ τῆς ἀφ᾽ ἡμῶν ἀποφερο-
μένης θερμότητος ἐγκαθιζούσης τοῖς
περιβολαίοις. * * καὶ μὴν ὅτι καὶ ὑγρότης ἀποφέρεται
πιστοῦσιν ἀπὸ τῶν ἱματίων· ξηρὰ γὰρ περιβαλόμενοι
ταῦτα καταλαμβάνομεν ἔνικμα γενόμενα διὰ
10 τὸ ὑγρόν, ὡς καὶ ὑγρότης ἐγκαθίζουσα ἡμῖν ἀποφέρεται ἀπὸ τῶν ἡμετέρων σωμάτων. οἱ γὰρ . . . . . .
κοι πρὸς ὄρθρον διαναστάντες . . . .
βαρυνόμενοι τῆς γινομένης . . σ . . . τυ . . . . . .
ορευγομενοι ταυ . . . .
15 μετὰ τὸ περιπάτωι . . . .
τροφῆς τινος γενηθεν . . . δι . . . .
πολλῶν διαπεφορημέν . ι . . . .
λόγωι θεωρητοὺς ἀπὸ τῶν ὑ . . . .
καὶ οὐ μόνον δὲ τοῦτο κατασκευάζουσιν, ἀλλὰ ὅτι
20 καὶ διάφοροι ἀποφοραὶ γίνονται ἀπὸ τῶν σωμάτων.
καὶ τοῦτο ὑπομιμνήσκουσιν οἱ περὶ Ἀσκληπιάδη
καὶ Ἀλέξανδρον τὸν Φιλαλήθη, ὅτι τὰ αἰσθητῶς κενούμενα διάφορά ἐστιν καὶ τὰ κατὰ τὸ λόγωι
θεωρητὸν ἀποφερόμενα οἷα . . . .
25 ὅτι δὲ τὰ αἰσθητῶς κενούμενα διάφορά
τέ ἐστιν καὶ ποικίλα, ὡς ἀπεδείξαμεν, δῆλον· ἔστι γὰρ ξηρὰ

XXXV. 11. Supply, says D., something like ὑδρωπικοὶ or ἄγροικοι.
14. P. reads ορευγομενοι. D. suggests ἐρευγόμενοι or ὀρεγόμενοι.

XXXIV the foods in us because these foods do not come under the cognizance of the sense. For just as that which is being digested must be in an appropriate place, if digestion is to take place, and just as what is changing into blood must be in an appropriate place if the change into blood is to occur, so too the object of smell must be in an appropriate place if smelling is to occur. And so these things that are in us, if they do not fall under the cognizance of a sense, naturally escape its notice. For this reason, when sweet-smelling things are taken, the sense does not apprehend the qualities of these things. Thus much in reply to

XXXV Asclepiades. * * they say too that there are given off from our bodies warmth and moisture. And that heat is given off they suggest by the following arguments. If we put round us our cloaks when they are rather cool, we find them warmer, which tends to show that the heat coming off us is absorbed by our coverings. * * And further, that moisture too is given off they try to prove from our cloaks. If we have put them round us when they are dry, we find that they have become humid through the moisture, which shows that moisture, being absorbed in us, is given off from our bodies. . . . .

. . . . And they not only maintain that this is so, but also that different kinds of emanation come off from our bodies.

33   The followers of Asclepiades and Alexander Philalethes also suggest that sensible evacuations are of different kinds, as are emanations to be inferred only by reason, e.g. . . . . . . Clearly, as we have proved, sensible emanations are different and various. For some are dry, some

---

XXXIV. 53.   The subject of λέγουσι and of ὑπομιμνήσκουσι (XXXV. 3) appears to be the Erasistrateans.

XXXV   καὶ ὑγρά. * * καὶ ἄλλη ἐστὶν διαφορὰ κατὰ τοὺς τόπους·
ἃ μὲν γὰρ διὰ σιάλων κενοῦται, ἃ δὲ διὰ ἀποπάτων,
ἃ δὲ διὰ μηνιαίων...............
30   ον, ἃ δὲ δι' ἱδρώτων, πάντα δὲ ἀπὸ διαφόρων τόπων.
καὶ ἐφ' ἑνὸς δὲ τούτων κατ' ἰδίαν ταὐτὸ ὑπολάβοις ἄν.
ἐπὶ γὰρ τῶν οὔρων ἃ μέν ἐστιν παχέ†ι†α, ἃ δὲ λεπτὰ μᾶλλον,
ἃ δὲ χολώδη καὶ ἃ μὲν προσδεχόμενα τοιάσδε ὑποστάσεις,
ἃ δὲ τοιάσδε, ἃ δὲ οὐδ' ὅλως ὑφιστάμενα, καὶ ἃ μὲν ἐπι-
35   νέφελά ἐστιν, ἃ δ' οὔ. * ὡς ὁμοίως δὲ καὶ ἐπὶ τῶν ξηρῶν.
τῶν κενουμένων γὰρ αμ....... γὰρ αὐτῶν αἰσθητῶς
κενούμενα διαφέροντά ἐστιν δι.....κατὰ τὸ
λόγωι θεωρητὸν ἀπενεχθήσεται....
ἀπενεχθήσεται. * * ἑπομένως δὲ τούτοις φασὶν καὶ τὰ αἴτια
40   διαφέροντα. καὶ τοῦτο σαφὲς ἐπὶ τῶν τε ὑγρῶν
καὶ ξηρῶν· τοῦτο δ' ἐπὶ τῶν ὑγρῶν.......
καὶ ποικίλα αὐτῶν, ὅτι καὶ δια.....ασ-
ται καὶ ποικίλα. * * καὶ μὴν ἀπὸ ...τ...ν
ἀποφορὰ γίνεται καὶ ἀπὸ γυ.ρ..υ ἀποφέρεται, διαφερόντως
45   δὲ καὶ ἀπὸ νεύρων, ὀστῶν, προσαι.....ένων.
εἴπερ δὲ καισ.αι ἀπ' αὐτῶν ἀποφοραὶ οὐκ..... γίνονται, εἴπερ
ἡ τροφὴ αἷμα. εἰ δὲ τοῦτο οὕτως ἔχει, καὶ ἀπὸ
μέρους διαφέρουσαν ἀποφορὰν....εἰν. * ἀπὸ
παντὸς δὲ μέρους γινόμεναι ἀποφοραὶ α...ισ....,
50   ὅπερ ἐστὶν ἀδύνατον .τον.............
ἂν γένοιντο..... γὰρ δυναμ....ων τ........
τοῦτο κατὰ τὴν φαντασίαν. * *..........
περὶ τὸ αἷμά τοι καὶ γενήσονται .ωσ..αι αυ.. αυ-
των τῶι καὶ κατ' Ἀλέξανδρον λόγωι ἐλέγχει τοῦτο

XXXVI   ὁπωσοῦν. οἷον γάρ, φησίν, ἔστι τὸ αἷμα κατὰ τὴν φαντασίαν,
τοιοῦτο καὶ κατὰ τὴν δύναμίν ἐστιν, ἁπλοῦν τι καὶ μονοειδές.
νωθρὸν δ' ἐστίν..υτα γὰρ ὀρθῶς ἔχει· καὶ γὰρ παρὰ
τὰς δυνάμεις ἐστὶν διάφορον τὸ αἷμα καὶ παρὰ
5   τὴν κατεργασίαν τῆς τροφῆς. * ταύτηι δὴ διάφορον

XXXV. 45–53.   The reconstruction of these lines is mere guesswork.
48.   After ἀποφορὰν we should probably supply ἔστιν (or ἦν) εὑρεῖν.
XXXVI. 1.   Perhaps φασίν.
3.   Perhaps τοῦτο οὐ γὰρ.
4.   τὴν δύναμιν K.   The terminations are illegible (or almost so) in P.

XXXV moist. * * There is also another kind of difference, depending upon

place. For there are evacuations of sputa, evacuations through the

bowels, menstrual evacuations...........................

...............evacuations through sweating, all of which come

from different places. And from one of these in particular the same

conclusions could be drawn. For in the case of urine, it is sometimes

thick, sometimes rather thin, sometimes bilious, sometimes forming

one kind of sediment, sometimes another kind, occasionally with no

sediment, sometimes being cloudy, sometimes being clear. * Similarly

too in the case of dry evacuations.......as may be inferred by reason

will emanate......will emanate. * * Conformably with these, they say,

the causes too differ. And this is clear in the case of both wet and

dry....... * * And moreover from......emanation occurs and ema-

nates from limbs (?) but in a different way from sinews also and

bones......But since...emanations from them do not......occur,

seeing that the nutriment is blood. And if that be so, a different emana-

tion from a member can be found. * But from every member emanations

taking place......which is impossible.......would prove......

this according to the appearance * * ......about the blood of course

will actually take place......by the reasoning of Alexander also

XXXVI somehow refutes this. For, he says, as blood is simple and uniform in

appearance, so it is simple and uniform in its properties. Stupid reasoning

this, not borne out by facts. For blood differs according to the properties,

and according to the digestion, of the nutriment. * It is just in this way

XXXVI   τὸ ἐπὶ τῶν ἀθλητῶν παρὰ τὸ ἐπὶ τῶν ἰδιωτῶν· τὸ μὲν γὰρ
λεπτότερόν ἐστιν, τὸ δὲ τῶν ἐναντίων παχύτερον.
ἐπεὶ δ᾽ οὖν διάφορόν ἐστιν τῶν ἐν ἡμῖν τὸ προκείμενον,
διάφοροι γένοιντ᾽ ἂν καὶ ἀπ᾽ αὐτοῦ αἱ ἀποφοραί. * *
10   ὅτι δὲ καὶ παρὰ τὴν τῆς τροφῆς κατεργασίαν διάφορον ἂν γένοιτο τὸ αἷμα καὶ ἑτεροῖον κατὰ τὰς δυνάμεις, οὐ
χρεία
πολυλογίας· ἡ γὰρ τροφὴ ληφθεῖσα πρώτης κατεργασίας
τυγχάνει ἐν στόματι καὶ διαφόρου γε ταύτης. εἰ μὲν γὰρ
μ.... λεαι....ηεισδησει μᾶλλον....ψιν τε
                                                        χ
15   καὶ ..ψιν ....επι....ν ἀπολεαιν.... κακο
αν κατασκευα.ει .... αἷμα καὶ τοὺς χυμοὺς
...... αιμ δι.. τοῦ φλέγματος ..περιέχειν
...τοῖς δὲ Ἐρασιστρατείοις τἄνπαλιν δοκεῖ ἄλλην ἐκεῖ
γίνεσθαι εἰκότως παρὰ τὴν ἐν τῶι στόματι κατεργασίαν. * *
20   διαφόρου γὰρ ὑπαρχούσης διάφορον κατασκευάζεται τὸ αἷμα
κατά τε δύναμιν
καὶ χρῶμα * ἐπεὶ τοιγάρτοι διάφορόν ἐστιν τὸ αἷμα, διάφοροι
καὶ κατὰ τὸ λόγωι θεωρητὸν ἀποφοραὶ ἀπ᾽ αὐτοῦ
γίνονται. * * καὶ παρὰ τὴν ἐν τῆι κοιλίαι δὲ κατεργασίαν διάφορον ἂν γένοιτο τὸ αἷμα· διὰ δὴ τοῦτο καὶ
25   διὰ κοιλίαν κένωσιν ποιῆσαι ἔστιν. * καὶ ἐπὶ τῶν ἄλλων
.....μάτων τοῦτ᾽ ἄν τις εἴποι· καὶ γὰρ παρὰ τὰς δια-
γωγὰς καὶ παρὰ τὰς φορὰς καὶ κεινήσεις διαφορὰς
τῶν ἀποφορῶν γίνεσθαι. * καὶ ἐπὶ δὲ τῶν ἄλλων σωμάτων,
ἀρτηριῶν
καὶ φλεβῶν καὶ ὑμένων κοινότερον εἰπεῖν διαφορὰν καταλείπουσιν,
30   ἢ αἰτία τῆς τούτων διαφορᾶς γενήσεται. * ὅτι δὲ·
καὶ κατὰ τὰς κεινήσεις διάφορα γίνεται τὰ σώματα,
φανερόν. οἱ γὰρ κινητικώτερον βιοῦντες
θερμότερα ἔχουσιν τὰ σώματα καὶ διὰ τοῦτο
πλείονα τὴν ἀποφοράν, οἱ δὲ ἰδιῶται τοὐναν-

---

13. ταύτης H. Schöne. Only -ς legible in P.
14. D. suggests εἰ μὲν γὰρ μὴ ἀπολεαίνεται, ἐκεῖ σχήσει μᾶλλον τὴν
ἔψιν τε καὶ πέψιν, εἰ δὲ ἐπὶ πλεῖον ἀπολεαίνεται, κακοχυμίαν ἂν κατα-
σκευάζοι κατὰ τὸ αἷμα καὶ τοὺς χυμοὺς λυμαίνοιτο διὰ τοῦ φλέγματος
τῶι περιέχειν αὐτό. For ἐκεῖ σχήσει read ἐπισχήσει.
26. διαιτημάτων or δὲ σωμάτων.

XXXVI that the diet of athletes differs from that of ordinary folk. For the one is poorer, that of the opposite class richer. Accordingly, as that of our constituents which is in question varies, the emanations too from it will be different. It requires little discussion to show that digestion of food also will produce varieties of blood differing from one another in their powers. For nutriment when taken undergoes its first process of digestion in the mouth, and this digestion differs from others. [For if nutriment be not softened, it will have its seething and digestion checked. But if it be over-softened, it may produce an unhealthy condition of the blood, and harm the humours through the phlegm by its surrounding them.] The followers of Erasistratus, on the other hand, are of opinion that there takes place in all probability a process of digestion there varying with that taking place in the mouth. * * For it is because the digestion is different that the blood produced is different in property and colour. * Since therefore the blood is different, the emanations too from it prove different to the eye of the reason. * * Furthermore, blood will prove different because of the digestion in the belly. It is for this reason too that it is possible to evacuate through the belly (?). * In the case of other bodies this can be said. For varying with modes of life, and with motions and movements differences of emanations occur. * And in the case too of the other bodies, they admit a variation of arteries, veins and membranes, to speak generally, which will prove to be the cause of the variations of these emanations. * And that on account of movements too bodies become different is clear. For those who live active lives have bodies that are warmer, and therefore give out a more copious emanation, while with ordinary folk the contrary holds good.

22. Hackforth would add αἱ after καί.
25. A rare sense of διά with accusative. See XXVIII. 13. Perhaps: "it is possible to adopt a low diet for the sake of the belly", i.e. the belly can be given a rest by taking food digested elsewhere. A lecturer's aside in either case.
26. According to another restoration "diets".

XXXVI 35   τίον. ταῦτα γὰρ παρὰ τὰς ὥρας τἀτὸ κατασκευάζουσιν

....τι....ι.ερεια διὰ τὴν ὑπέρμετρον θερμασίαν

....μεν ....ροι πλεῖον κενοις τῶι

λεπτυνόμενα τὰ παρακείμενα καὶ ῥευστικὰ

γινόμενα κενοῦσθαι κατά τε τὸ αἰσθητὸν

40   καὶ κατὰ τὸ λόγωι θεωρητόν · * * κατὰ μέντοι γε τὸν χειμῶ-

να ἧσσον. * ἐκ τούτων τοιγάρτοι φανερόν, ὡς

.... μὲν αἱ ἀποφοραὶ κατὰ τὸ λόγωι θεωρητόν

.... οὗται. ὥσπερ δὲ κατὰ τὸ λόγωι θεωρητὸν

καὶ κατὰ τὸ αἰσθητὸν διάφορα καὶ ποικίλα ἀποκρίνεται

45   ἀφ᾽ ἡμῶν, οὕτως καὶ κατὰ τὸ αἰσθητὸν εἰσκρίνεται

διάφορα εἰς ἡμᾶς καὶ κατὰ τὸ λόγωι θεωρητόν,

ἅπερ τετόπασται καὶ πρότερον, καὶ Ἀσκληπιάδης

διά τινος ὑπομνήσεως τοιαύτης · ἡ φύσις, φησίν,

τηρητικὴ καθέστηκεν τοῦ τε δικαίου καὶ

50   τοῦ ἀκουλούθου. ἐπεὶ γὰρ ἀπεκρίνετό τινα κατὰ τὸ

αἰσθητόν, ὡς ἐδείχθη, καὶ κατὰ τὸ λόγωι θεωρητὸν

δέδοκται καλῶς, ὡς καὶ τοῦτο κατεσκευάκαμεν, τὸν

αὐτὸν τρόπον καὶ κατὰ τὸ λόγωι θεωρητὸν καὶ

κατὰ τὸ αἰσθητὸν διάφορα εἰσκριθήσεται εἰς

55   ἡμᾶς. * * καὶ ὅτι μὲν εἰσκριθήσεταί τινα κατὰ τὸ λόγωι

θεωρητόν

εἰς ἡμᾶς, πρῶτον ἀπὸ τῶν δυνάμεων τῶν

κατὰ τὰ φάρμακα ἔξεστι σκοπεῖν, * καιατῶν ἢ

καπνῶν καὶ καταπλασμοῦ, ἃ ἐπιτιθέμενα

XXXVII   τῆι ἐπιφανείαι ὁτὲ μὲν διαλύει τὰ ὑποκείμενα,

ὁτὲ δὲ διαφορεῖ, ἄλλοτε δὲ ἐπισπᾶται. τίνος

γινομένου; οὐ μόνον τῆς δυνάμεως αἰτίας ὑπαρχούσης τῶν

φαρμάκων

τῆι ἐπιφανείαι προσκαθιζούσης, ἀλλὰ καὶ εἰς βάθος

5   ἄχρι του αἰτίας διοδευούσης διὰ τῶν λόγωι θεωρητῶν

πόρων τοῦ σώματος. * ἐξ ὧν φανερόν, ὡς καὶ κατὰ

τὸ λόγωι θεωρητὸν εἴσκρισις γίνεται εἰς ἡμᾶς. * καὶ μὴν

καὶ κατὰ τὸ αἰσθητὸν εἴσκρισις γίνεται. ὃ γὰρ τὸ ἐλα-

τήριον εἰσκρινόμενον εἰς τὸ σῶμα ποιεῖ†ν†, τὸ

XXXVI. 36.   Perhaps ὃ τὰ λοιπὰ ἐν θερείᾳ (D.)

37.   D. suggests τότε μὲν γὰρ οἱ πόροι πλεῖον κενοῦσι τῶι.

43.   "Sensus: διάφορα δὲ κενοῦται" D.

XXXVI Athletes sweat more owing to the seasons than others do in summer with its excessive heat.................For then the passages exude more, because their contents becoming refined and liquefied are voided both to sense and to the eye of the reason. * * in winter however less. *

34 From this therefore it is plain that the emanations are different to the eye of the reason, and different things are evacuated. Just as both to the eye of the reason and to sense different and varied emanations come from us, so to sense and to the eye of the reason different accretions penetrate into us, as has been conjectured before, and as Asclepiades says, in some such remark as this: "Nature habitually preserves law and consistency." For since certain secretions were taking place, sensible as was shown, and since other invisible emanations have been rightly judged to occur, as this too we have established, in the same way both to the eye of the reason and to sense different accretions will penetrate into us. * * And that certain accretions, perceived by the eye of the reason, will penetrate into us, we may first illustrate from the strong qualities of drugs * of mints or of fumitories and of plaster,

XXXVII which being placed on the surface sometimes dissolve what lies under it, sometimes dissipate it in perspiration, and sometimes draw it to themselves. What happens to cause this? The cause is that the strong quality of the drugs not only settles on the surface, but also penetrates down to a certain depth through the passages of the body that are to be apprehended by reason only. * From this evidence it is plain that penetration takes place into us that can be apprehended only by reason. * Furthermore sensible penetration also takes place. The same effect for example produced by the Purge when taken internally is also caused by external applica-

XXXVII 10 αὐτὸ καὶ ἔξωθεν ἐπιτιθέμενον ἐργάζεται.
καὶ εἰσκρινόμενον μὲν καὶ ἄνω καὶ κάτω καθαίρει ὑδατώδη τε καὶ χολώδη καὶ πᾶν τὸ παρ' ἄλλων.
διὸ καὶ δοκεῖ ἐνεργέστατον παντὸς καθαρτικὸν εἶναι
τὸ ἐλατήριον. ἕκαστον μὲν γὰρ τῶν καθαρτικῶν
15 ἕν τι ἀποτελεῖ ἀποτετελεσμένον, τοῦτο δὲ πάντα
ὅσα καὶ τἆλλα· καὶ γὰρ αλλεισι..α..ου ληφθὲν
οἷον ἡμιωβέλιον. * * ὁ μὲν οὖν ἐλλέβορος χολώδη καθαίρειν· καὶ ὁ μὲν λευκὸς ἄνω κεινεῖν,
ὁ δὲ μέλας κάτω καὶ τὰ σκαμώνεια ὑδα-
20 τώδη καθαίρειν. ἐκ τούτων τοιγάρτοι καὶ τῶν τούτοις
παραπλησίων φανερόν, ὡς τὰ μὲν ἄλλα τὰ προκείμενα ἕν τι δύναται, τὸ δὲ ἐλατήριον
πολλά. ἀλλὰ γὰρ καὶ ἔξωθεν ἐπιτιθέμενον τά-
τὰ δύναται· ἀναληφθέν τε καὶ ἀπὸ ῥινῶν ἢ καὶ ἐπι-
25 τεθὲν ἐπὶ τοὺς τῶν νηπίων ὀμφαλοὺς ὁτὲ μὲν ἄνω
καθαίρει ὁτὲ δὲ κάτω, καὶ νῦν μὲν χολώδη, νῦν
δὲ ὑδατώδη. τίνος γινομένου; δῆλον ὅτι
τῆς δυνάμεως τῆς κατὰ ταῦτα διικνουμένης
ἄχρι τῶν ὑγρῶν τούτων διὰ τῶν λόγωι θεωρητῶν πόρων.
30 καὶ μὴν καὶ ὁ λευκὸς ἐλλέβορος ἀποθυμιώμεν-
ος γυναιξὶ ἀγωγὸς γίνεται τῶν καταμηνίων διὰ τὴν
αὐτὴν αἰτίαν. * * εἶτα καὶ οἱ εἰλυσπώμενοι καὶ κα-
τα†λε†λυομένας ἔχοντες τὰς δυνάμεις
ῥώννυνται ταύτας οσ.... ἄρτων... ὀδμαί * κἀνταῦ-
35 θά φησιν, ὡς λόγος ἔχει, Δημόκριτον ἀσιτήσαντα
τέσσαρας ἡμέρας πρὸς τῶι ἀναιρεῖσθαι γίνεσθαι·
καὶ αὐτὸν παρακληθέντα πρός τινων γυναικῶν
ἐπιμεῖναι ἡμέρας τινὰς ἐν τῶι βίωι, ἵνα

---

35. Laertius Diogenes, IX. 43: τελευτῆσαι δὲ τὸν Δημόκριτόν φησιν
Ἕρμιππος τοῦτον τὸν τρόπον. ἤδη ὑπέργηρων ὄντα πρὸς τῷ κατα-
στρέφειν εἶναι· τὴν οὖν ἀδελφὴν λυπεῖσθαι, ὅτι ἐν τῇ τῶν Θεσμοφορίων
ἑορτῇ μέλλοι τεθνήξεσθαι καὶ τῇ θεῷ τὸ καθῆκον αὐτὴ οὐ ποιήσειν.
τὸν δὲ θαρρεῖν εἰπεῖν καὶ κελεῦσαι αὐτῷ προσφέρειν ἄρτους θερμοὺς
ὁσημέραι. τούτους δὴ ταῖς ῥισὶ προσφέρων διεκράτησεν αὐτὸν τὴν ἑορτήν.
ἐπειδὴ δὲ παρῆλθον αἱ ἡμέραι (τρεῖς δὲ ἦσαν), ἀλυπότατα τὸν βίον προή-
κατο. Caelius Aurelianus, acut. morb. II. 37 (p. 166 Amman): sit igitur polenta
infusa atque panis assus aceto infusus vel mala cydonia aut myrta et his similia.
hae enim defectu extinctam corporis fortitudinem retinent, sicut ratio probat atque
Democriti dilatae mortis exemplum fama vulgatum.

---

38. τινας D: τέσσαρας K.

XXXVII tion. When taken internally it clears away both by the mouth and by stool watery and bilious matters, and every morbid element from other humours. Wherefore too the Purge is acknowledged to be the most effective cleanser from every humour. For each of the cleansing medicines accomplishes one definite object, but this achieves all that is done by all the others. In fact half an obol when taken is sufficient. * * Now hellebore clears away bilious matters; the white evacuates by vomiting, the black by stool. Scammony clears away watery matters. Therefore from this and similar evidence it is plain that the drugs under consideration have one particular power, but the Purge has many. In fact even external application of it has the same result. Taken in by the nostrils or placed upon the navels of infants it purges sometimes by vomit and sometimes by stool, now bilious matters, now watery matters. What happens to cause this? Clearly the power in these respects reaches as far as these moist matters through the passages that are apprehended by reason. Furthermore white hellebore used in fumigation promotes menstruation in women for the same reason. * * Then too people who are prostrate and have their powers decayed are strengthened if they take in the smell of loaves. * On this matter Asclepiades says that, according to the story, Democritus having fasted for four days was near to death. Certain women besought him to remain in life a few days longer, so as to prevent their suffering the ill-

14. The "Purge" was the juice of the wild cucumber, used for a variety of purposes. See Celsus, v. 12 and Pliny, xx. 1–3.
18, 20. The construction of the infinitives is obscure.
32. εἰλυσπώμενοι means literally, "crawling".

XXXVII   μὴ γένωνται ταύταις δυστυχῶς τὰ κατὰ
40   κείνους τοὺς χρόνους Θεσμοφόρια λελυ-
μένα, φασὶν αὐτὸν ἀπαλλάττειν κελεῦσαι, καθείζειν δὲ πρὸς τοὺς
ἄρτους, καὶ τούτους καταπνεῖν ἀτμὸν τὸν
γινόμενον †δουδημοκριτο†. καὶ ὁ Δημόκριτος ἀπο-
σπασάμενος τὸν ἀπὸ τοῦ ἱπνοῦ ἀτμὸν ῥών-
45   νυταί τε τὰς δυνάμεις [καὶ ἐπιβιοῖ τὸ] λοι-
πόν. ἐπεί τε ὑδάτια†ν† καὶ τὴν λειμὸν κορέννυσιν
καὶ οὕτως διεξαρκ[εῖ, δῆλον ἂν εἴ]ποιμεν, ὡς
καὶ διὰ τῶν λόγωι θεωρητῶν πόρων ἡ αἴσθησις
γίνεται εἰς ἡμᾶς. * * καὶ ἀπὸ τῶν ἐπιφανειῶν †εις†
50   τοῖς ἡμετέροις σώμασι προσφέρεται τὸ προστεθέν †μενον†.
καὶ γὰρ, φησίν, τὸ καστόρειον προστιθέμενον τοῖς
μυκτῆρσιν ἐνίοτε ῥώννυσι τὰς δυνάμεις διικνουμένης τῆς ἀπὸ τοῦ καστορείου δυνάμεως διὰ τῶν λόγωι
θεωρητῶν
καὶ ἐντεινούσης. * * τούτωι γέ τοι προσβάλλων
55   ὁ Ἀσκληπιάδης κατασκευάζει, ὡς οὐ παρὰ τὸ κατατάσσεσθαι τὸν ἀτμὸν ἀπὸ τῶν ἄρτων
ταῖς δυνάμεσι ῥώννυνται ταύτας, ἀλλὰ
παρὰ τὸ διεγείρεσθαι τὴν ψυχήν. * ὅνπερ

XXXVIII   γὰρ τρόπον τὸ καστόρειον προσοισθὲν τοῖς μυκτῆρσι
ῥώννυσι τὰς δυνάμεις διεγεῖρον τὴν ψυχὴν καὶ ἐν-
τεῖνον, τὸν αὐτὸν καὶ οἱ ἀτμοὶ γινόμενοι.
ἀλλὰ τοὐναντίον· τὸ μὲν καστόρειον, ὥσπερ εἶπον,
5   ῥώννυσιν τὰς δυνάμεις διεγεῖρον τὴν ψυχήν, οἱ δὲ ἀτμοὶ
οὐ διεγείροντες τὴν ψυχὴν ὠφελοῦσιν, ἀλλὰ προσκατα-
τασσόμενοι τοῖς σώμασιν. * * γελοῖος δ᾽ ἐστὶν ἀνήρ·
οὐ γάρ, εἰ ἀμφότερα τὰ βοηθήματα διεγείρει τὰς δυνάμεις,
ταύτηι κωλυθήσεται τὸ ἕτερον προσκατατάσσεσθαι
10   τῶι σώματι. καὶ γὰρ δὴ ὁ τιλμὸς διεγείρει τὰς δυνάμεις καὶ
αἱ πληγαί, ἀλλὰ οὐχ ὁμοίως· διὰ μὲν γὰρ τῶν πληγῶν
καὶ τιλμῶν διεγείρονται αἱ δυνάμεις καὶ φυλάσσουσι
τὰ ἐν τῶι σώματι καὶ οὐχὶ ἐῶσιν ἀφανίζεσθαι,
ἀλλὰ πυκνώσεως γινομένης τηρητικαὶ
15   γίνονται τοῦ τε πνεύματος καὶ τῆς θερμότητος·

XXXVII. 47. "διεξαρκεῖ supplevi, ignotum lexicis, at notum Philoni I.
607 M" (D.).
48. αἴσθησις P.: εἴσκρισις Kalbfleisch.

XXXVII luck to have the Thesmophoria cancelled, that occurred at that season. They say he bade them remove him, and set him in the bakery, where the loaves shed over him the steam that arose. Democritus having inhaled the steam from the oven strengthened his powers and lived out his life. Since watery matters satisfy even hunger and so suffice, we could state as proved that sensation comes to us through the passages also that can be apprehended only by reason * * * and from the surfaces that which has been applied is added to our bodies. In fact, he says, castor applied to the nostrils sometimes strengthens the powers, the power from the castor penetrating with a bracing effect through the passages apprehended by reason. * * However, discussing this point Asclepiades maintains that the steam from the loaves strengthens the powers, not by absorption into them but by stimulating the

XXXVIII soul. * For just as castor applied to the nostrils strengthens the powers, by stimulating and bracing the soul, so too acts the steam coming from the loaves. But the reverse is the case. Castor, as I have said, strengthens the powers by stimulating the soul, but the steams are helpful, not by stimulating the soul but by being absorbed into our bodies. * *

35 But the man is ridiculous. It does not follow, if both these remedies stimulate the powers, that therefore one or other will be prevented from being absorbed into the body. For surely plucking and blows stimulate the powers, but not in a way similar to the vapours. * For through blows and pluckings the powers are stimulated and guard the contents of the body, not allowing them to disappear, but, owing to the compression that occurs, proving preservers of the breath and of the heat. But when

XXXVII. 48. Perhaps we should read εἴσκρισις ("penetration") for αἴσθησις.
XXXVIII. 10. τιλμός and πληγαί apparently refer to some kind of massage.

XXXVIII ὑπὸ δὲ τοῦ καστορείου καὶ τῶν ὁμοίων ῥωννύμεναι
αἱ δυνάμεις ὡς πρὸς τὴν ὀσμὴν τὸ αὐτὸ ἐνεργοῦσι, * * ὑπὸ
μέντοι γε τῶν ἀτμῶν ῥωννύμεναι αἱ δυνάμεις καὶ
προστρεφόμεναι προσανακύπτουσιν. * δῆλον
20   τοιγάρτοι, ὡς ἀπὸ τῶν ἀτμῶν ῥώννυνται αἱ δυνάμεις
ἀφικνουμένων τῶν ἀτμῶν διὰ τῶν λόγωι θεωρητῶν
πόρων, ἐξ ὧν ὁμολογουμένως κατασκευάζουσιν,
ὡς καὶ εἰσκρίνεταί τινα εἰς ἡμᾶς διὰ τῶν λόγωι
θεωρητῶν πόρων τῆς σαρκός. * * ἄλλως τε ζητεῖται,
25   πῶς θερμαίνεται ἡμῶν τὰ σώματα · δῆλον γὰρ
ὡς τῆς θερμασίας εἰσκρινομένης εἰς τὰ ἡμέτερα
σώματα καὶ ἀλεαινομένων πρὸς αὐτῆς. εἰ δὲ εἰσκρίνεταί τις θερμασία εἰς ἡμᾶς, πῶς δῆτα εἰσκρίνεται;
σῶμα γὰρ αὕτη, σῶμα δὲ διὰ σώματος οὐκ εἰσ-
30   κρίνεται. οὐκοῦν διά τινων εὐρυχωριῶν; * εἰ τοῦτο,
πόρους τοιγάρτοι χρῆν ἀπολιπεῖν λόγωι θεωρητούς,
δι' ὧν εἰσκριθήσεται ἡ θερμασία. * ἐχομένως, φησίν,
καὶ ἐπὶ τοῦ χειμῶνος ψυχρότερα ἡμῶν ἐστιν τὰ
σώματα †το† τῶι τὸν ἀέρα ψυχρὸν ὄντα καὶ
35   εἰσιόντα εἰς ἡμᾶς καταψύχειν ἡμᾶς. * ταύτηι
γέ τοι ἐπὶ τούτων διαπορεῖται, τί δήποτε οἱ ἐκ τῶν
βαλανείων ἐξερχόμενοι καὶ ὑπὸ τῶι ἀέρι γενόμενοι
εὐθέως καταψύχονται, * οἱ μέντοι γε μετὰ τὸ λουτρὸν
περιχεάμενοι ψυχρῶι ἐν τῶι βαλανείωι, εἶτα
40   ἐν τῆι αἰθρίαι γενόμενοι ἧττον καταψύχονται.
τίνος γενηθέντος; δῆλον ὅτι τῆς μὲν καταχύ-
σεως τοῦ ψυχροῦ πυκνούσης τὴν ἐπιφάνειαν
καὶ κωλυούσης ἀφανίζεσθαι τὸ ἐν ἡμῖν θερμόν,
τόν τε ἀέρα ψυχρὸν ὄντα μὴ ἐώσης εἰσκρίνεσθαι.
45   διὰ δὴ τοῦτο τὸ αἴτιον μὴ ῥαδίως καταψύχεσθαι
τοὺς ποταμούς. * ἐπὰν μέντοι γε τοῦτο μὴ γένηται, ἀλλ' ἡραιωμένοι χωρήσωσι εἰς τὸν ἀέρα,
θᾶττον δέχονται αὐτόν, καὶ ὃς εἰσιὼν
εἰς τὰ σώματα ψυχρὸς ὢν καταψύχει αὐτά.
50   εἰ δὲ τοῦτο, φανερόν, ὡς εἰσκρίνεταί τι ἀπὸ τοῦ

---

45. Read καταψύχειν, as several scholars suggest, or perhaps τοῖς
ποταμοῖς.
48. ὃς: ὡς (?) Hackforth.

XXXVIII strengthened by castor and such like, the powers produce the same effect on the sense of smell, * * * * by vapours however the powers while strengthened are also nourished and refreshed as well. * It is clear therefore that from vapours the powers are strengthened, the vapours reaching them through the passages manifest to reason only; from which facts they make the incontestable inference that there is also penetration into us along the passages through our flesh that are manifest to reason only. * *

36 Another question arises: how are our bodies heated? For it is clear that it is through the heat penetrating into our bodies, which are warmed by it. But if a sort of heat penetrates our bodies, how, one asks, does it do so? For heat is body, and body does not penetrate through body. Is it then through certain free spaces? * If so, then it is necessary to postulate passages manifest only to reason, through which heat will penetrate. * Agreeably to this, Asclepiades says, our bodies are colder in winter, because the cold air enters and chills us. * At this point, however, a difficulty arises in the matter. Why, we ask, is it that those who come out of the bath are at once chilled on reaching the air * but those who after washing pour cold water over themselves in the bath, are less chilled on coming into the open air? What has happened? Clearly pouring cold water contracts the skin and prevents the heat in us from disappearing, and does not allow the cold air to penetrate. It is just for this reason that rivers too do not easily cool us. * When however this has not been done, and men go into the air with the pores open, they receive it quicker, and because it is cold when it enters our bodies, it cools them. If that be so, it is plain that something from the air

45. For μή see p. 33.

XXXVIII   ἀέρος εἰς ἡμᾶς. * * διδάσκουσι δὲ καὶ μετὰ ταῦτα, ὡς εἰσίν τινες λόγωι θεωρητοὶ πόροι
ἐν τοῖς ἡμετέροις σώμασιν, ὅπερ δή ἐστιν γελοῖον.
πρῶτον μὲν γὰρ ἐχρῆν τοῦτο κατασκευάσαι καὶ τοῦ-
5   το προκαταστησαμένους λοιπὸν διδάσκειν,
ὅτι καὶ ἀποκρίνεταί τινα ἀπ' αὐτῶν διάφορα, ὡς
ὁμοίως δὲ καὶ εἰσκρίνεται, ὃ οὐ δοκεῖ γίνεσθαι.
τοῦτο ᾱ. ἀλλὰ δεύτερον δι' ἦν αἰτίαν..........
ἀλλ' αυτη . ατιτα......................

XXXIX   θαι Ἀλέξανδρος, προσχρῶνται. καὶ ᾱ, φησίν, ἀποκρίνεταί τινα ἀφ' ἡμῶν καὶ εἰσκρίνεταί τινα εἰς
ἡμᾶς πάντως διά τινων λόγωι θεωρητῶν πόρων,
ἐπειδήπερ σῶμα διὰ σώματος οὐ λέγουσι διελθεῖν.
5   καὶ ἄλλως φησίν· ὡς ἡ φύσις τηρεῖ τὸν νόμον, ἐποίησεν
πάντων ἀποφοράς τινας αἰσθητὰς καὶ λόγωι θεωρητάς
καὶ διαφόρους ἀποφορὰς κατὰ τὸ αἰσθητὸν καὶ κατὰ τὸ
λόγωι θεωρητόν. * ἐπεὶ οὖν κατὰ τὸ αἰσθητὸν
ἐποίησέν τινας πόρους, καὶ κατὰ τὸ λόγωι θεωρητὸν
10   ἐποιήσατο, * ὅτι τρέφεται, φησίν, πάντα διὰ πόρων
τοῦ σώματος καὶ οὐ λέγουσιν σῶμα διὰ σώματος
διελθεῖν, καὶ τὸ χυλωτὸν καὶ τἄλλα τοῦ σώματος
μέρη γίνεται τῆς τροφῆς διοδευούσης .αι..
..........ος μέρος τοῦ σώματος, ὡς τῶν
15   λόγωι θεωρητῶν πόρων ὄντων ταύτῃ ...
.. ὁ Ἐρασίστρατος θαυμάζει ἐπ...ι...των
..ληται τὰ τηλικαῦτα λ..σφε.αι....
κατακαέντα ὑφ' ὑάλου καὶ ει.......
..ε κατὰ τοῦτον ἁπλοῦν αὐ.......ειεν
20   ..ον.......... τήγανον καὶ .....ον
διαφοραὶ ..ς φυσ...ς μὲν ἐχειταιδημε...ς
αὐτοῖς λόγωι θεωρητοὺς πόρους .....εν καὶ

XXXVIII. 52.   Sextus Empir. adv. math. VIII. 220: Ἀσκληπιάδῃ δὲ ὡς
ἐνστάσεως νοητῶν ὄγκων ἐν νοητοῖς ἀραιώμασιν (rubor cet. signa
videntur).

XXXIX. 1.   D. says that the sense is: τῇ αἰτίᾳ ᾗ καὶ Ἀσκληπιάδῃ
φησὶν χρῆσθαι.
10.   ἐποίησε τᾱτό H. Schöne: ποιησάτω D.
15.   Perhaps a full stop should be placed after ὄντων.
18.   καὶ εἴλης H. Schöne.

XXXVIII penetrates into us. * * The followers of Asclepiades maintain, after this, that there are certain passages in our bodies to be apprehended by reason. This is surely absurd. This they should have proved first, and then, after establishing the point, they should have gone on to maintain that various things emanate from the pores, and similarly too penetrate through them, which latter is not thought to take place. This is the first point. Secondly, they adopt the explanation of causation which Alexander

XXXIX attributes to Asclepiades.......... First, he says, certain things emanate from us and penetrate into us without doubt through certain passages apprehended by reason, since body, they say, cannot pass through body. And besides, he says also: As nature maintains uniformity, he postulated from all bodies emanations, both sensible and also apprehended by reason only, and emanations differing according to sense and also according to the apprehension of reason. * Since then he postulated certain passages apprehended by sense, he also postulated the same postulate about passages apprehended by reason, * because all things are nourished, he says, through passages of the body (and they deny that body passes through body), and the fluid becomes the other parts of the body also as nourishment passes through ...showing that the passages apprehended by reason exist.... Erasistratus wonders....burnt by a burning-glass or sun heat....frying pan...nature gave to all animals the same kind of passages

XXXVIII. 51. The subject of διδάσκουσι is the followers of Asclepiades.
XXXIX. 1. The conjectural emendation of D. is adopted.
5. The subject of ἐποίησεν is perhaps ἡ φύσις. This is confirmed by l. 25. So ll. 9 and 10.
10. The reading of Schöne is adopted.

XXXIX

ἡμῖν. ὡς γὰρ καὶ μύρμηξ τρέφεται, οὕτως
καὶ ἐλέφας καὶ αἱ Βακτριαναὶ κάμηλοι ἂν
25 τραφεῖεν τῶι τὴν φύσιν καὶ ἐπὶ τούτων πάντων πόρους τινὰς καὶ κατὰ τὸ αἰσθητὸν καὶ
κατὰ τὸ λόγωι θεωρητὸν μεμηχανῆσθαι,
ἵνα καὶ τὰ ἐλάχιστα τῶν μερῶν τρέφηται
τῆς τροφῆς διικνουμένης ἐπ᾽ αὐτά. φανερὸν
30 τοιγάρτοι ἐκ τούτων καὶ τῶν τούτοις παραπλησίων, ὡς λόγωι θεωρητοὶ πόροι εἰσὶν ἐν ἡμῖν
καὶ παντὶ ζώιωι.

ANONYMI LONDINENSIS

FRAGMENTVM

οἱ γὰρ προθυμίαι γινόμενοι πρὸς τὸ διαχωρῆσαι,
καταλαμβανόμενοι δὲ ἐν ἀγορᾶι ἢ
ἐν ἀνεπιτηδείοις, εἶτα συσχόν-
τες ἐπὶ πλεῖον, οὐκέτι διαχωροῦσιν
5 ἢ διαχωροῦσιν ἐλάχιστά τε καὶ ξηρά.
τίνος αἰτίας γινομένης; δῆλον ὅτι ἀποφορᾶς καὶ ἐντὸς
ἀπ᾽ αὐτῶν γεγενημένης. ἐξ ὧν φανερόν,
ὡς τροφή ἐστιν καὶ ἡ ἐν ἐντέροις παρακειμένη. * * ἐὰν δέχῃ τούτων οὕτως ἐχόντων

Fr. I. 8.   Caelius Aurelianus, *acut. morb.* I. 14 (p. 44 Amman): *praeterea
excrementa ventris (Graeci σκύβαλα dicunt) negat* [Asclepiades] *aliena esse
natura, si quidem etiam ex ipsis corpora augeantur.*

---

32.   P ends with the argument unfinished. This fragment is the largest
of several on the back of the papyrus.

XXXIX apprehended by reason that she gave to us. For as an ant is nourished, so too elephants and Bactrian camels would be nourished through the fact that nature has in the case of all these constructed certain passages, both sensible and also apprehended by reason, in order that even the least of the parts may be nourished as nourishment passes through to them. Therefore it is clear from this and such like evidence that there are passages apprehended by reason in us and in every animal.

FRAGMENT

Those who are anxious to go to stool when seized in the market-place or in other unsuitable places, should they restrain themselves for any length of time, either do not go to stool or pass a very small, dry motion. What is the cause? Clearly because inside us also emanation from them has taken place. Wherefore it is plain that nutrition extends also along the bowels.[1] * * If you admit, these things being so,.....

---

[1] "Or is it ἡ ἐν ἐντέροις παρακειμένη (ἀποφορὰ) τροφή ἐστιν?" Cornford. This is perhaps more probable.

EXCURSUS I

THE NATURE OF GREEK THOUGHT

This brief description of Greek thought is not intended to be a full account of the subject. All that has been attempted is to bring into relief that aspect of philosophy which appears in medical theories set forth in many parts of the Hippocratic *Corpus* and in the second section of *Anonymus*.

For φιλοσοφία is indefinite in its meaning and strange in its character. Under the term was included every activity of the mind, from theological speculation to elementary grammar, although of course various thinkers would tend to lay stress on the importance of one branch of knowledge or to demand the exclusion of others. Perhaps the remark of Plato,[1] repeated by Aristotle,[2] that philosophy began in curiosity, gives, better than any formal definition, the essential characteristic of all Greek thought. The spirit of disinterested research, working for the sheer love of knowledge without any utilitarian motives, is the one factor common to Greek philosophy throughout the period during which it flourished. In many departments this spirit, in itself a great contribution to human progress, achieved results of much value. In ethics, logic and psychology, and later, when the natural sciences were better understood, in the biology of animals and of plants, the foundations were laid upon which, with certain radical changes of outlook and method, later thinkers reared the superstructure of modern science.

The subjects mentioned in the last paragraph deal with phenomena (γιγνόμενα), with the effects of reality (ὄντα) upon our consciousness and powers of perception. But right from the birth of philosophy Greek thinkers felt, consciously or unconsciously, that φιλοσοφία was, in a special sense, concerned with ὄντα and not with γιγνόμενα. In modern phraseology it meant metaphysics, and the sciences had a claim to the name only in so far as they were dealt with in a philosophic spirit, and with an effort to discover their relations to the reality underlying them. Mere sequences of phenomena, the formulation of which satisfies many modern workers in the field of scientific research, gave

---

[1] *Theaetetus*, 155 d. [2] *Metaphysics*, A 2, 982 b.

but little satisfaction to a Greek. Nevertheless, in a secondary and looser sense, the name of "philosopher" was not always refused to a thinker of a less spiritual order, provided that he was serious and thorough, presenting his subject in an orderly, systematic way. The title was even claimed by the shallow educationist Isocrates, in direct opposition to the philosophic idealist Plato. It may conduce to clearness if "thought" and "thinker" be used as far as possible when speaking of philosophy in its wider, looser sense.

This brief sketch of the scope of Greek philosophy has led us to consider its aim—the pursuit of knowledge for its own sake. Such a motive is, of course, a potent factor in modern research, but it is perhaps less powerful than the urge to harness Nature to our service by the discovery of natural processes. So Macaulay was not very far wrong when in his brilliant essay on Francis Bacon he maintained that the old philosophy was one of words, the new philosophy one of works, the one discussing undiscoverable ultimates, the other seeking to invent new conveniences for the use of suffering mankind. Greek culture, it has been well said, is a strong protest against the view that the chief object in life is to make men more comfortable. It strove after the eternal verities, and up to a point was one with Christianity in laying stress upon the spiritual side of man.

In spite of the vagueness and uncertainty that obscure the conception of φιλοσοφία, the Greek view of its aim and purpose is quite intelligible, and receives sympathetic appreciation to-day from a large number of thoughtful people. But the case is far otherwise when we examine its actual pronouncements, and the methods by which these conclusions were reached. These are often strange and perplexing, not to say startling. What are we to think when Empedocles [1] declares, confidently and dogmatically, that bone consists of two parts of water, two of earth and four of fire? Assuming that Empedocles was trying to express the inner truth of things, are we to take his statement literally? If not, what did he mean by it? By what methods was the formula discovered? One wonders, too, what answer Empedocles would have given to an opponent who urged that the proportions of the elements were wrong, or that another set of elements should have been chosen, or that the so-called elements were not elemental. One could put similar questions to Anaxagoras, and inquire on what grounds, and with what purpose, he declared that blood, bone and marrow were elements, but that air and water were not. Practically the whole of

[1] Quoted by Aristotle, de anima, 410a.

Plato's *Timaeus*[1] consists of a fantastic cosmology followed by an equally fantastic physiology, without any proofs that a modern scientist would accept for a moment, and with but the flimsiest reasons assigned for its explanations, dogmatically expressed, of the most obscure mysteries. Turning to the philosophy of medicine and the views held by the highest authorities about the origins of disease, we meet with the same confident dogmatism, the same superficial reasoning, the same ignoring of obvious objections, and the same lack of caution and discipline before accepting a generalisation. The medical students whose opinions are given in the *Anonymus Londinensis* seem to think that dogmas such as "All diseases are due to excess of one of the four humours", or that "Most illnesses are caused by residues of food", have only to be enunciated to be believed. In fact many, if not most, of the fundamental theories of Greek philosophers appear to be largely guesswork.

One may naturally wonder whether it is possible to explain to modern minds, if only in part, the strange nature of Greek thought. Perhaps it is quite impossible for one generation to understand the mentality of another, however much care is given to the difficult task of a just appreciation. Though hard, the task must be attempted; to shirk it is to misunderstand a great part of extant Greek literature. Of the reasons that suggest themselves as at least partially responsible for the great difference between ancient thought and modern, the first to be considered, though possibly not the most powerful, is the extreme youth of the intellectual movement which, beginning in Ionia about six hundred years before Christ, was most active during the fifth century and the earlier part of the fourth. The early Greek philosophers were the pioneers of rational thinking, and the fifth century B.C. saw but the infancy of Greek thought. Curiously enough, although it may be a mere coincidence, child psychology presents some close analogies to the efforts of fifth-century Greeks to answer the questions that presented themselves to their minds. The child, like the Greek, loves to guess, and is intolerant of slow and cautious methods. Again, both love the world of imagination, and are disposed to prefer artistic truth to philosophic or scientific truth, should it ever be necessary to make a definite choice between them. The unfinished picture annoys the child as it annoyed the Greek, who filled it in by the art of the poet and the romancer whenever gaps occurred that otherwise must have been left

---

[1] Plato indeed says (*Tim.* 29 d and 59 d) that he is giving but a plausible and probable account. But he expresses himself positively, and in dogmatic language, while his main thesis, that the Demiurge created the Universe and Man in the best possible way, is as dogmatic a ὑπόθεσις as any in Greek philosophy.

as blank spaces, because the philosopher had no material to work upon. The most striking examples of this use of fiction are the "myths" in Plato's dialogues. When everything has been done permitted by the nature of things to the Intellect, then, but not till then, Fiction comes to the aid of Truth and fills in the missing detail.

The Greek, again, resembled the child in his instinct to begin with the organised whole rather than with the separate and individual parts. When studying a new language the child must start with the sentence, and not the parts of speech; and in a similar manner Thales, at the birth of Greek philosophy about 600 B.C., speculating about the "stuff" out of which the Universe is composed, declared it to be water and nothing but water; nearly two hundred years were to elapse before Leucippus and Democritus conceived of atoms, not unlike the chemical atoms of fifty years ago, as the elemental constituents of the physical Universe.

This childish, uncritical attitude in speculative thought was encouraged, rather than checked, by the absence of utilitarian motives. When to-day a theory is born out of a desire to improve the condition of human beings, it is at once subjected to the strictest and most severe of tests—"Will it work?" Unless some concrete, practical results follow the acceptance of this theory, it is condemned and rejected without delay. The utilitarian aim, in fact, acts as a brake, and a most efficient one, on all rash theories and hasty generalisations. These flourish and run riot whenever there is no incentive to test their usefulness, and to measure their truth by their success when applied to the problems facing mankind in the physical world. The preacher who makes wild statements about heaven arouses little opposition and perhaps little interest, and so rash theological guesses are not rare, but the analytical chemist who tries to persuade a brewer to base the making of beer upon a random guess is asking for trouble. That a theory must work before it can be entertained is a commonplace of modern science. An ancient theory did not need to "work" at all, because no such usefulness was expected of it. Critics required that it should be rational; they did not require that it should produce tangible results.[1]

The strangeness, however, of Greek philosophy and thought was not entirely due to its youth. Many other influences were acting upon

[1] See the interesting passage in Xenophon, *Memorabilia*, i. i. Though the objections to contemporary philosophy are put into the mouth of Socrates, they are really those of the philistines of the day, who desired something more "useful" than philosophical speculation. The rise of so-called "Sophistry" was due to the same desire to substitute vocational for purely cultural education.

it, difficult to appreciate, and more difficult still to weigh and arrange in their order of importance.

In the first place, we must remember that philosophy preserves considerable traces of the cosmogonies, or accounts of the creation of the world, which immediately preceded it. When we read about Anaximander's "Boundless",[1] and how the world evolved itself out of it, we are reminded of chaos, "without form and void", and of the creation therefrom of the heavens and ordered Universe. The mental atmosphere of this teacher's work, indeed of all philosophy down to (and possibly including) the Atomists, is that of poetry or religious faith, rather than that of "science", although superstition has been superseded by rational, if not plausibly reasonable, arguments and explanations.

A suggestion has recently been made[2] that many of the wilder guesses of Greek thinkers were similar in spirit to our intellectual games. It is a fact that the human mind has an almost irresistible urge to indulge the imagination without the restrictions imposed by appeals to sense experience. Moderns delight in fiction of all sorts, seeking to escape from the workaday world, and to lose themselves in the world of romance. We read novels or visit the cinema; we play games demanding intellectual alertness, such as chess or cross-word puzzles. In this way we seek recreation, and at the same time make our minds supple and ready for the serious business of life. But in the case of us moderns, our spheres of recreation are outside and apart from our serious work. The physician does not "play" at medicine, but at golf or bridge; the chemist does not "play" at formulae, but at tennis or perhaps football pools. In other words, a sensible man has a hobby, and however seriously he takes it, he allows himself a freedom in its pursuit that he dare not allow in carrying on his profession. To this general rule there are a few exceptions serving to prove it. The Rev. Edwin A. Abbott wrote *Flatland, A Romance of Many Dimensions by a Square*, and occasionally a physicist will indulge his imagination in describing the "mysterious" Universe. But the ancient philosopher rarely had a hobby, and his mental recreations were few and unsatisfying. So he was thrown back upon his serious occupation to find recreation and amusement, and appears to have seen nothing incongruous in intro-

---

[1] The ἄπειρον was a mass, perhaps infinite in amount and certainly undifferentiated in quality, a kind of mist or cloud, from which the famous "opposites", now first heard of, separated themselves out.

[2] "The Scientist's Playground", by W. H. S. Jones, in the *Proceedings of the Royal Society of Medicine* for February 1937.

ducing sportive speculation into places where to our minds strictly
scientific reasoning alone is admissible. The Number in Plato's *Republic*
is an obvious instance, and the "play-hypothesis" may perhaps explain
more of the strangeness of Greek thought than can be proved, or than
scholars are ready to admit.[1] Of course the "play" was subject to the
rules of the game, which were logical consistency and adherence to
artistic truth. The Greek liked a "true story" even when he could not
have a "really true story". In mediaeval days thinkers found a playground for their games in theology. Here the rules were very strict,
and a violation of them might mean death at the stake.

The spirit, however, animating the greater part of Greek philosophy
is not that of play. Down to Aristotle, with few exceptions, the mood
of the writers is what may not unfairly be described as devout. The
religious instinct of the Greeks had few means of expressing itself
except through the channels of sculpture, architecture and tragedy.
They had no Bible, in our sense of that term, and so the intellectual
side of religion, the application of belief to every-day problems, became
the concern of philosophers. Theological speculation, too, was merely
a part of physics or metaphysics; a Greek had nothing to correspond
to our creeds, articles of religion and Church doctrine. So Greek
thinkers showed a keen interest in a world removed from our senses,
where "faith vanished into sight" and knowledge was perfect and
complete. Plato consistently refuses to call ἐπιστήμη almost everything that a modern scientist would call "knowledge", the Platonic
name for all this being "opinion" (δόξα). Much, then, that cannot be
proved by the strict canons of scientific method was accepted by Greek
thought because it gave not irrational answers to many questionings
of the human mind, although these answers involved a definite act
of faith. We are not surprised to find that the sphere of faith was often
extended to departments of philosophy to which it is not applicable.
"Medicine has no need", says the writer of *Ancient Medicine*,[2] "of
an empty postulate, as do insoluble mysteries about which any exponent
must use a postulate, for example, things in the sky or under the earth."
The mistake to which the author refers is one we often meet in the
history of Greek thought, and especially in the history of the medical
sciences.

---

[1] See especially *Timaeus*, 59 d: "When a man, for the sake of recreation, lays
aside discourse about eternal things and gains an innocent pleasure from the
consideration of such plausible accounts of becoming, he will add to his life a
sober and sensible pastime" (Cornford's tr.).

[2] [Hippocrates], περὶ ἀρχαίης ἰητρικῆς, 1. 1.

This yearning after perfect exactness and positive assurance was strengthened, and at the same time more closely determined, by several subsidiary factors, of which, perhaps, the most influential was the successful study of geometry[1] and kindred studies by the Greeks generally, and by Pythagoras and his school in particular, before Greek thought cast its swaddling clothes. Now geometry was considered, and to a great extent is, an exact science, and so are all branches of pure mathematics. It starts with rigid postulates, axioms, and definitions, and proceeds to equally rigid and precise conclusions. Words like "nearly", "apparently", "perhaps", "approximately", are entirely out of place in its demonstrations. "Equal" in geometry means exactly equal, not approximately so. The Greek thinker, trained in a mathematical school, felt, with Plato, that all knowledge ought to possess similar exactitude, without any of the indefiniteness similar to that which is inseparable from all graphic representations of lines, triangles and circles. Hence the scepticism, apparent in Greek thought from Xenophanes and Heraclitus, about the value to be attached to the evidence of the senses. Over the door leading to Plato's lecture-room was the inscription, "No admittance for those who have not passed through the course of geometry", and in the *Republic* he makes mathematics an indispensable preliminary to the study of dialectic, or philosophy proper.

Thus Greek philosophy has a mathematical as well as a theological bias. As geometry is a deductive science, proceeding from accepted premises to logically necessary conclusions, so Greek thought shows a strong tendency to follow a similar method, even when induction is the natural, or the only possible method. It usually begins with a postulate (ἀρχή, ὑπόθεσις) or postulates, on which is built up an elaborate superstructure, which stands or falls with the security of the foundations. The dogma of Thales, "All things are water", that of Parmenides, "The ent is, the non-ent is not", and that of Plato, "Besides phenomena that become, there are Forms that really are", are all unproved assumptions,[2] dogmatically asserted as self-evident truths.

---

[1] Geometry ("earth-measurement") developed earlier and more rapidly than other branches of mathematics, which awaited the invention of a simple system of notation. "Geometry" often means in Greek all mathematical studies then known, while the Pythagorean "numbers" seem to have been points and figures, plane or solid. Students of conic sections, algebraical and geometrical, will readily appreciate the Greek tendency to look at mathematics from a geometrical standpoint.

[2] Hebrew thought, too, as expressed in the Old Testament, has a deductive bent, its premises being the will of God revealed in the Law and the Prophets.

In fact most philosophic "hypotheses" are attempts to pierce the veil that shuts off reality from our senses, and as such cannot be tested and judged by the same canons as are used to-day to confirm or reject a scientific theory. The latter does not pretend to go beyond secondary causes; the former were attempts, however unsuccessful, however pathetically inadequate, to find a first principle and a primary cause. Though a Greek expected the logical consequences of a philosophical hypothesis to agree roughly with sense-experience, yet he would never have admitted[1] that a theory must be incorrect if inconsistent with one observed phenomenon. He would have thought it possible, even probable, that the phenomenon harboured some deception that our senses cannot detect.

It is therefore not to be wondered at that Greek thought pays little attention to the collection of evidence, and still less to the method of experiment. There are, of course, a few well-known experiments described by philosophers, and there is a fair sprinkling in the works of the Hippocratic *Collection*.[2] They are, however, only the exceptions that prove the rule, and they occur in those parts of Greek thought that approach nearest to the modern sciences. A mentality nurtured in its early education on mathematics and metaphysics naturally had a great predilection for the methods of these subjects, and an equally great distrust of the senses, carrying these prejudices into regions of thought where sensations are the material out of which an organised science has to be built up. The quick-witted Greek seems to have preferred a rational guess to a legitimate deduction from carefully collected evidence.

It will be plain from what has been said that the Greeks realised the difference between "knowledge" and "opinion" earlier and more easily than they did the difference between the methods by which they can be attained. The result was a long controversy between philosophers and scientists, both sides defending their respective "ways of inquiry", and the philosophers, on the whole, had the advantage in the struggle. The triumph of philosophy was due in great part to the logical acumen of Parmenides, who argued cogently that truth cannot come through the senses but must be apprehended by pure intellect. What our brains tell us must be true, and if our senses tell us one thing and our brains another, so much the worse for the senses. The dictates of the intellect, which according to Parmenides express the

---

[1] Epicurus, with his ἀντιμαρτύρησις, is possibly an exception.
[2] These have been discussed by G. Senn in Sudhoff's *Archiv für Geschichte der Medizin* (1929), pp. 217–288, in an article entitled "Ueber Herkunft und Stil der Beschreibungen von Experimenten im Corpus Hippocraticum".

truth about reality, are of the nature of axioms or postulates. Such intuitive apprehension of reality was considered to be a part, perhaps the chief part, of what the Greeks called θεωρία, "looking on as a spectator", which Aristotle[1] asserts to be the activity peculiar to God, and shared by men in so far as men partake in the divine nature.

So throughout the history of Greek thought the twofold conflict goes on. The methods appropriate to θεωρία are imposed upon the study of phenomena; students of phenomena hold that their researches and conclusions ought to contribute something to θεωρία. In other words, there is being made an effort to discover the right relation between philosophy (ἐπιστήμη) and the sciences (τέχναι). In this conflict a most important part was played by the τέχνη of medicine.[2]

---

[1] Aristotle, *Ethics*, x. 8 (1178b).
[2] See especially Professor Heidel's recent work *Hippocratic Medicine*.

EXCURSUS II

THE NATURE OF GREEK MEDICINE

Of all the sciences, medicine is the most likely to develop and assert itself in the early history of any nation. It arises out of imperious human needs, being controlled at every point by the equally imperious necessity of meeting these human needs. Unless it works cures it is discredited. Of course, disease is associated even to-day with superstition and irrational credulity; in early Greece such superstition was far more prevalent. In Homer the view is held that sickness comes from a god, being therefore unavoidable.[1] Superstitious treatment, such as amulets and incantations, found favour with the many, and the writer of the famous *Sacred Disease* is at great pains to prove that there is nothing "divine" in epilepsy or fits. The point needs no elaboration, such superstition being universal in primitive societies. What is more, sick folk in all ages are likely, under the nervous prostration of illness, to take refuge in quack remedies and superstitious devices, not so much because they distrust scientific medicine, as because fear makes them catch at straws and revert to the primitive impulses of their savage ancestors.

But, however much patients may be prone to superstition, medical practitioners begin to be rational in all societies that have emerged from barbarism, just because scientific treatment, if such be known, obviously pays; while as civilisation progresses rational medicine establishes itself, taking control of new areas, consolidating its conquests, and gradually growing in popular favour.

The triumph of reason over unreason was far more certain and rapid in Greece than it appears to have been in other countries. The "medicine-man" or super-quack has few if any representatives, Empedocles being a doubtful claimant of a more than doubtful honour. Even in Homer surgery and physic are crafts, based, empirically no doubt, on reason, and when after Homer the light at last pierces the darkness that envelops the centuries down to 500 B.C., we find rational medicine securely established, with rival schools, each with its own principles of diagnosis, methods of treatment, and theories about the aetiology of disease.

[1] See *Odyssey*, IX. 411.

Between quacks and scientific physicians came two classes of practitioners—the priests of the temples of healing and the physical trainers.

The temples of Asclepius, a curious blend of Lourdes and rest-cure homes, were under the management of priests who added a little medical lore to a profound knowledge of the mentality of half-educated hypochondriacs. Most of the cures effected by them were the outcome of healthy surroundings and cleverly-staged "suggestion". Usually the patient after a rest of varying length was made to sleep in the sacred precincts of the Asclepieum, where the god was supposed to visit him in a dream, the nature of which indicated the line of treatment to be adopted. The priests professed to interpret these dreams, demanding from those who improved in health a fee with a testimonial or advertisement of their skill. Several of these advertisements have been discovered on two pillars in the temple of Asclepius at Epidaurus. They present a striking contrast to the famous forty-two clinical histories to be found in the First and Third Books of *Epidemics*; the one is a series of miraculous cures, the other of scientific studies of cases which usually end in death. It is now realised by medical historians that temple-healing, as practised by the priests of Asclepius, can have contributed little or nothing to legitimate medicine.[1]

Outside, but only just outside the circle of regular practitioners, were the physical trainers and gymnastic instructors, who followed a profession respected throughout all Greece. It was their business to keep men healthy by adjusting exercise to diet and diet to exercise. In fact, the ablest Greek physicians agreed that medicine was, in essentials, merely a branch or modification of the science of dietetics. A most interesting treatise (*Regimen*) in the Hippocratic *Corpus* was written—not for athletes but for ordinary folk[2]—by one of these trainers, who not only gives elaborate rules, based on an ingenious theory, for the preservation of health, but claims that by modifying regimen most diseases can be checked if discovered in good time. So far as is known, this is the earliest work dealing with preventive medicine.

In order to appreciate Greek medicine correctly we must understand something about the conditions in which the physician worked. In

[1] There is no reference in the Hippocratic *Corpus* to any such connection.
[2] The first chapter of the treatise *Affections* (περὶ παθῶν) asserts that the ἰδιώτης ought to have some medical knowledge, in order to co-operate with the physician, and the author proceeds to give it. It is strange that the discussion begins with the ὑπόθεσις that all diseases are caused by excess of the dry, the moist, the hot or the cold acting on bile and phlegm.

the first place, it appears likely that infectious diseases were rare, or had not yet found a home in Greece. Typhus and bubonic plague probably visited Mediterranean countries at long intervals, but the Hippocratic *Collection* contains no sure and certain descriptions of diphtheria, scarlatina, small-pox, measles, chicken-pox, or even influenza. There are a few cases that may possibly be the first, and many historians take it for granted that typhoid is included among the types of sub-continuous fevers (καῦσος, etc.) that are so common in all the Greek medical writings. The difficulty of diagnosis lies in the possibility of explaining the syndromes of symptoms in various ways, while typhoid (if present) is so mixed up with malaria in the accounts of καῦσος and similar fevers that, in the absence of epidemics or even of single cases that can be typhoid and nothing else, it is safer to infer that such cases were remittent malaria. This was endemic in the Greek world, and is often so like typhoid that only the microscope can distinguish between them. Mumps[1] is described once, not as an endemic disease, but as an unfamiliar nameless epidemic attacking Thasos towards the close of the fifth century B.C. So far as is known, the Greek medical writers never refer to it again. The endemic diseases of ancient Greece can be reduced almost entirely to two groups—chest complaints and malaria. Pleurisy, pneumonia and pulmonary tuberculosis were rife; the Greek even knew that phthisis was infectious,[2] while the physician's familiarity with pneumonia was such that he knew when and how to operate for empyema. Malaria, both intermittent and remittent, was so common that it was often called simply "fever" without further qualification. A remark, significant in more senses than one, occurs in Greek literature, to the effect that fevers are not infectious.[3] Malaria *is* infectious, although not conveyed by touch or breath. A Greek would naturally infer that it was not infectious, but how such a remark could be made by anyone familiar with measles, influenza or typhoid it is difficult indeed to see. The common types of disease being only two, it was not unnatural that many doctors tried to reduce the causes of at least acute diseases to one, and to treat all such in much the same way.

If medicine had a limited sphere of action, it had also a very limited supply of aids to therapeutics. A Greek physician had no thermometer, no stethoscope, no microscope, no antiseptics, no chemical

[1] Hippocrates, *Epidemics*, I. i.
[2] See e.g. [Aristotle], *Problems*, VII. 8, and Isocrates, *Aegineticus*, 29, where the patient is suffering from φθόη (§ 11).
[3] [Aristotle], *Problems*, VII. 8.

reagents. He was perhaps fortunate in having few drugs and no very strong inclination to use even these few, but he was sadly handicapped in having no trained nurses. When skilled nursing seemed called for, he left one of his pupils[1] in charge. These apprentices, as we should call them, acquired in this way the experience a modern medical student acquires by walking the hospitals. The nursing in less serious cases, or when a pupil was not available, fell to the slaves and women[2] of the household, but the physician does not seem to have regarded their help with approval.[3]

In such conditions, and with these handicaps, it is not surprising that the Greek love of restraint and moderation showed itself clearly in the practice of the Greek physicians. They promised their patients very little, and avoided heroic treatment. The best of them[4] adopted the simplest methods. If the patient was able to get about, gentle remedies might be tried, such as dieting, baths, massage and easy exercises. The exercises, if we may take those given in *Regimen* as a fair example, often show a striking likeness to those used for training recruits in the war of 1914–1918, while the baths resemble our Turkish or Russian baths. Serious cases were sent to bed and kept quiet, a radical change of diet being imposed. In the diet of the sick, barley-water was the great stand-by. There still survives a longish work, possibly from the hand of Hippocrates himself, called *Regimen in Acute Diseases*, containing instructions for the preparation and use of this food, from the thinnest gruel to the thickest porridge, with rules for its administration. Wine and honey, the latter often mixed with vinegar or water, were sometimes prescribed, plain water and milk being used less often than they are to-day. Baths, fomentations, enemas, suppositories, and a few drugs, the last being chiefly purgatives, made up the physician's equipment. Emetics the Greek doctor appears to have regarded as quite as useful, if not more so, than purges acting on the bowels.

Before the significance of pulses was understood, fever, in the absence of thermometers, was measured by the touch. It is indeed strange that in the Hippocratic age physicians did not use the pulse as a means of diagnosis. Although they knew that pulses existed, they did not

---

[1] [Hippocrates], *Decorum*, XVII.
[2] Xenophon, *Oeconomicus*, VII. 37.
[3] *Decorum*, loc. cit.
[4] Methods of treatment naturally varied, and, as time went on, drugs came more and more into use. The means of healing mentioned in this paragraph are taken from the Hippocratic *Corpus*.

appreciate their medical significance till the end of the fourth century B.C. Galen, of course, had a full knowledge of pulses.

The training of medical students is difficult to describe in a brief sketch, as it probably varied from time to time, and at no period is our information other than scanty in the extreme. We could speak more positively did we know more about the medical "schools". Herodotus[1] tells us that of these the earliest flourished at Croton and Cyrene; before the end of the fifth century there had come into prominence the schools of Sicily, Cnidos and Cos. But we know nothing about the organisation of any of these schools, nor is it clear that they had any organisation, in the modern sense of the term. We must certainly clear our minds, if we wish to understand pre-Alexandrine medicine, of all modern ideas associated with universities, professors and elaborately staffed hospitals. The nearest modern, or rather mediaeval, equivalent to ancient conditions is the guild. Whatever may be the date of its final form, the Hippocratic Oath seems to represent, at least in outline, the status of the medical student during the fifth and fourth centuries B.C., as the Platonic evidence[2] is strongly in favour of such a conclusion. In other words, the usual relation was that of apprentice to master, not that of undergraduate to professor. In many cases, though probably not in all, the master travelled from city to city[3] as did the Sophists, taking his apprentices with him, and employing them as assistants and nurses.

This close personal contact with an experienced master insured the practical nature of the student's training, while travel probably brought an experience as varied as that provided by modern hospitals. But there would be a tendency for master-physicians to associate themselves with places, which became the homes of physicians of pre-eminent ability and reputation. In this way Euryphon founded the school of Cnidos, and Hippocrates that of Cos. There were thus formed societies of physicians with more or less definite, and perhaps peculiar, views, though it is quite impossible to gauge the degree of cohesion among the members of each society. Equally vague is the relation between these societies and the super-guild of the Asclepiadae. From the time

[1] III. 131.
[2] See Protagoras, 311 b, where a young man, wishing to become a professional physician, is said to be likely to put himself under Ἱπποκράτη τὸν Κῷον, τὸν τῶν Ἀσκληπιαδῶν.
[3] The first part of Airs Waters Places was written to help such περιοδευταί, as they were called, and to place at their disposal some collective experience of the effects of climatic conditions upon health and disease. Decorum too appears to assume that travelling physicians were common.

of Theognis[1] a medical man was, by courtesy at least, styled an Ascle-piad, just as to-day all qualified practitioners are styled "doctors".

But there was also, though it had ceased to exist, so far as we can see, before the time of Galen, an exclusive family of physicians, who claimed descent from Asclepius and taught their sons practical anatomy, trans-mitting their knowledge orally.[2] After a time, according to Galen, these Asclepiadae began to take pupils from outside, who transmitted the art much less perfectly. The relation of the Asclepiadae to the priests of Asclepius is also a doubtful question, although modern opinion[3] is tending towards the view that there was no connection between them.

In Alexandrine and post-Alexandrine times arose many sects or schools of thought—for such were most Greek medical schools—Empirics, Methodists and so on, but during the fifth century B.C. two schools competed for leadership, those of Cnidos and Cos, and these must claim our immediate attention. A third, however, the Sicilian-Italian school, which flourished at the same time or earlier, had perhaps more influence upon philosophic thought, its chief members being Alcmaeon, Empedocles and Philistion.

The Cnidians took a mechanical view of diseases, attaching great importance to the study of them as separate and individual entities. So they classified them with careful, not to say elaborate, attention, special stress being laid upon correct diagnosis. Galen[4] tells us that they recognised four diseases of the kidneys, three kinds of tetanus and three kinds of phthisis.[5]

The first three chapters of *Regimen in Acute Diseases* contain a criticism of the treatise *Cnidian Sentences*[6] (Κνίδιαι γνῶμαι), supposed to have been written by Euryphon, the founder of the school. The writer admits[7] that "the later revisers have shown rather more scien-tific insight" than was shown in the first edition, but blames the

---

[1] LI. 432–434.
[2] Galen, II. 281. Cf. Plato, *Laws*, IV. 720: τούς τε αὐτῶν διδάσκουσι παῖδας. Other references are Galen, X. 4; XIII. 273; XIV. 676; Plato, *Republic*, 405 c and 406. *Protagoras*, 311 b; Lucian, *Lexiphanes*, 4.
[3] See E. T. Withington, *Medical History*, pp. 45, 46, 378 and his excursus in W. H. S. Jones' *Malaria and Greek History*, pp. 137–156.
[4] XV. 427, 428.
[5] This agrees with *Internal Affections* (Littré, VII. 188–210). See also Galen, XVII. A 888 for a close parallel between a passage in *Diseases*, II, 48, and *Cnidian Sentences*.
[6] One cannot help feeling that these three chapters, whatever their origin, are no part of the main work, which begins at Chapter V. The fourth chapter is con-nected neither with Cnidian doctrine nor yet with regimen; it merely insists on the need of showing thoroughness and correctness in medical practice.
[7] Ch. III.

Cnidians generally on three different counts. They attached, it is alleged, too little importance to prognosis, and too much to the discussion of unessential details; their treatment was faulty,[1] and the number of remedies employed by them[2] was far too small; they carried the classification of diseases to extremes, holding that a difference in symptoms necessarily implied a different disease.

Many treatises in the *Corpus*[3] show Cnidian tendencies; in some cases, such as *Diseases* II and *Internal Affections*, the influence is strong, in others, for example the gynaecological books, it seems weaker. From these facts it may be inferred that Cnidian doctrine had its effect on physicians who did not fully belong to the school, and in fact on medicine generally. Its contribution to medical thought was to emphasise the truth that diseases are separate objective realities, external to the constitution of the patient. In the long run this view resulted in the discovery of bacteria, although it remained for centuries a dim, ineffective notion. Littré[4] urges that Cnidian medicine reached its full development in the nineteenth century A.D. It is interesting to note that if we confine our attentions to the more practical works in the *Corpus*, the greater number lean to the Cnidian, rather than the Coan, school of thought. For example, the gynaecological books, as we have said, belong to the former. The Cnidian books are text-books to help the physician on his rounds, and lay most stress on diagnosis and prescriptions.

The writer of *Regimen in Acute Diseases* complains that the Cnidians neglected prognosis. The term does not mean now quite what it meant in the fifth century B.C., when it was far wider and more comprehensive. "Prognosis" included, besides the forecasting of the future, the discovery from present symptoms what the past has been. It is in fact full acquaintance with the natural history of the "case", implying that the physician can infer from (1) his judgment of the patient's constitution and (2) his experience of the disease in others, what the whole of this particular case-history has been and will be.

It is not easy to understand why the Coan physician should have disparaged diagnosis, which to-day is thought to be of the first importance. It was perhaps due to his conviction that the resemblance

---

[1] We have a specimen in the treatment of pus in the lung: "drawing out the tongue they thrust into the trachea something moist of a kind to produce a violent fit of coughing" (Galen, I. 128, 130).

[2] They were purges, whey and milk.

[3] Ermerins makes a formidable list. See his *Hippocrates*, III. viii.

[4] *Hippocrates*, II. 200–205.

of all "acute" diseases to one another was essential, while their differences were unimportant, "diseases" in fact being merged, after the Platonic method, in "disease". We may more easily see why prognosis, which in its narrow sense is now thought to be comparatively unimportant, was valued so highly. In the absence of degrees and diplomas it helped a physician to gain the confidence of his patient by telling him what his previous symptoms had been, as well as by correctly forecasting the future. The foundation of this simple therapeutic and practice was an equally simple theory. The genuine Hippocratic looked upon an illness as a sort of battle (ἀγών) between the constitution (φύσις) of the patient and a morbid state generally regarded as a disturbance in the equilibrium of the constituents[1] of the human body. This battle had a natural course, including critical days, variation from which was unusual and alarming, and a major crisis. At this crisis the issue of recovery or death was decided. If it was to be recovery, there gradually took place a restitution of the equilibrium of the constituents, any residue being evacuated, either through the normal channels or by an ἀπόστασις, which may perhaps be rendered "abscession". Examples are abscesses, rashes and eruptions of all kinds. The chief duty of the physician was to watch this ἀγών as a very interested spectator, and to remove as far as possible all obstacles to the efforts of the patient's constitution, with its naturae vis medicatrix, to overcome the disease.

This dynamic conception of disease is to-day gradually returning to favour. There is, in fact, perennial value in the conception that the constitution of the patient is a factor to be taken into account no less than the morbid element. An illness is caused, not so much by a microbe as by the patient's defective reaction to it. Bettering the constitution is at least as important as destroying micro-organisms. Equally valuable is the conception that treatment should be mainly to put the patient in a state of repose, to task his bodily functions as little as possible, and to conserve his strength, so that the vis medicatrix may fight out the battle with the best possible chance of a speedy success.

The strict Coan seems to have almost confined his activities to applying these simple rules and theories to his medical practice. But there were others, some perhaps not practitioners, who held that medicine had much to learn from philosophy and its inquiry into the

---

[1] The Coans held that these were the four "humours", blood, phlegm, black bile and yellow bile. Other physicians took some of these humours with perhaps others, while the Sicilian-Italian school, followed by Plato, took as components the four "elements", earth, water, air, fire. See pp. 19, 81.

ultimate nature of the physical universe. They hoped to do for medicine of their day something analogous to that which modern chemists are doing for modern physicians. There are in the Hippocratic *Corpus* several works in which attempts are made to impose upon medicine the views of philosophers and their method of postulates. There is also one,[1] a book showing wonderful insight and power of thought, in which such attempts are vigorously resisted. Medicine in its turn had some effect upon philosophy, for there were physician-philosophers who at least subconsciously realised that there were inter-relations between the two.[2] It is this speculative theory that appears so prominently in the second section of *Anonymus*, in which are collected the opinions of physicians and of philosophers about the origins of disease. The Greeks liked to indulge their constructive imagination in this way, pouring out suggestion after suggestion in great profusion. Such speculation is far from useless if it keeps to its proper sphere, and does not encroach upon practical theory. The classic instance is Sir Patrick Manson's guess that malaria and mosquitoes are connected, which led to the epoch-making discovery of Sir Ronald Ross. Unfortunately the Greeks had not the tools to sift their guesses and to turn the happy ones into scientific truths.

So down to at least 400 B.C. we find medicine and physical philosophy influencing each other. At some time after this date, probably within Plato's lifetime, a change took place. Medicine, especially after the classification work of Aristotle, kept within its own borders, having little to give to physical science and little to receive from it. Physicians speculated, but confined their speculation more or less to their own subject. Without borrowing they worked at what may be called the metaphysics of medicine. After Aristotle we find medical practice more modified by theoretical speculation than it was before him. The Methodists, for example, based their therapeutic on a fantastic theory of constriction and relaxation of the πόροι in the body. But this theory was, as it were, autogenous; it owed little or nothing to the stream of genuine philosophic thought. So in a sense "medicine was separated from philosophy".

[1] *Ancient Medicine.* When Celsus in his Preface says that Hippocrates "separated medicine from philosophy", he probably was thinking less of this book (which, had he known it, he would doubtless have attributed to Hippocrates) than of the general character of Hippocratic medicine.

[2] There were many who realised that to understand the body one must understand the universe of which the body is a part.

INDEX OF *NOTABILIA*

The edition of Diels has an index of Greek words. The *Introduction* to this edition (pp. 14–16) has an alphabetical list of names with notes.